"I dare you to read *Green Vanilla Tea* and not fall in love with this family. Marie Williams has written a beautiful memoir about facing illness and loss with love and hope. She has opened her family's life and experiences to us in a way that will help us stay in touch with the richness of life and relationships, even in times of heartbreak and the loss of dreams. Thank you, Marie Williams, for this extraordinary love story."

> —**Jill Freedman, MSW**, family therapist and director of
> Evanston Family Therapy Center in Evanston, Illinois,
> as well as coauthor of *Symbol, Story, and Ceremony*;
> *Narrative Therapy*; and *Narrative Therapy with Couples*

"This beautifully written memoir of a husband and father who suffers a premature death is also a story about how families and communities cope with the ambiguous loss that precedes the physical death of a loved one. In the words of a young child who was part of the nurturing community that surrounded Dominic, 'we will crowd you with our love.' Insightful, heart-rending, and inspiring, this book offers the details of a family's life shattered by Dom's years of decline and death from a rare neurological condition. While particular about these people, *Green Vanilla Tea* provides lessons about love, care, generosity, and sadness. With unflinching descriptions of the darkness and despair the family faced, the book also shows their path toward solace and hope. Movingly, it shows how they were able to repair and restore a sense of wholeness to their interrupted lives. I highly recommend this brave book."

> —**Kaethe Weingarten, PhD**, associate clinical
> professor of psychology at Harvard Medical School
> (1981-2013) and director of the Witnessing Project
> at www.witnessingproject.org

D1007167

"Heartbreaking, compelling, warm and compassionate. It's a knockout book that hits so many of the right notes and is completely relevant in today's world. And it's unbelievably—considering the tragedy—uplifting. An inspiring read."

—**Susan Duncan**, author of *Salvation Creek*

"[I was] moved by the tragedy of the story, and the love and trust and care and kindness everybody showed."

—**Jacqui Kent**, editor and author of *The Making of Julia Gillard*

"Nobody has the right to have the last word on a book as beautiful as this. There would be few who have loved and cared for a person with dementia who will not be able to relate to the many moments of acute sadness, laughter, and joy in this book."

—**Ita Buttrose, AO, OBE**

"*Green Vanilla Tea* is the winner of the 2013 Finch Memoir Prize and it's easy to see why. Williams has written a powerful and heartbreaking account of her husband's illness, and the challenges faced by the family, which never loses sight of the immense love that binds this family together. This is an inspiring and important memoir."

—**Sarina Gale,** Books + Publishing

"The standard of the entries we receive improves every year. Marie won against some fierce competition including finalist Heath Lander's book *The Bouncer*, which we will publish later in 2013. However, the judges agreed that *Green Vanilla Tea* was the standout entry this year, making us laugh, cry, and above all, reflect on the value of love and family."

—**Rex Finch,** Finch Publishing

Green Vanilla Tea

*One family's extraordinary journey
of love, hope, and remembering*

Marie Williams

New Harbinger Publications, Inc.

Publisher's Note

"Living Memory" by Brian Andreas © 2012 Brian Andreas / Storypeople. Reprinted with permission.

Lyrics to "In Her Eyes" © 2006 Molly Kaye, Jeff Cohen, Michael Ochs, and Jeff Selby. Reprinted with permission.

Distributed in Canada by Raincoast Books

Copyright © 2014 by Marie Williams
New Harbinger Publications, Inc.
5674 Shattuck Avenue
Oakland, CA 94609
www.newharbinger.com

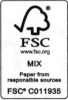
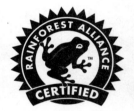

Cover design by Amy Shoup
Acquired by Tesilya Hanauer
Edited by Clancy Drake

Library of Congress Cataloging-in-Publication Data

Williams, Marie.
  Green vanilla tea : one family's extraordinary journey of love, hope, and remembering / Marie Williams.
      pages cm
  Includes bibliographical references.
  ISBN 978-1-62625-197-7 (paperback) -- ISBN 978-1-62625-198-4 (pdf e-book) -- ISBN 978-1-62625-199-1 (epub) 1. Williams, Marie. 2. Presenile dementia--Patients--Biography. 3. Presenile dementia--Patients--Family relationships. 4. Amyotrophic lateral sclerosis--Patients--Biography. 5. Amyotrophic lateral sclerosis--Patients--Family relationships. I. Title.
  RC522.W55 2014
  616.8'30092--dc23
  [B]

                              2014016204

Printed in the United States of America

16   15   14

10   9   8   7   6   5   4   3   2   1   First printing

To my sons—with all my love.

Living Memory

I carry you with me into the world
Into the smell of the rain
And the words that dance between people
And for me it will always be this way
Walking in the light
Remembering being alive together

—Brian Andreas, StoryPeople

Acknowledgments

I am deeply grateful to everyone who cojourneyed with us over the time of this story and beyond. Any thanks I offer here feels inadequate, but I hope that in our shared lives I have been able to let each of you know what a difference you made.

A special thanks to my beautiful family—for everything—I simply could not have done this without you.

To Pippa, my oldest friend, who read every evolving draft and offered me the greatest gift of listening.

To my friend and mentor Nike Sulway, for helping me polish this story for the boys and for believing in it so much, and for gently nudging me to release it to the world.

To the team at New Harbinger, for your enthusiastic support in bringing the North American edition to life.

And to the team at Finch Publishing—Rex Finch, Samantha Miles, and my editor, Laura Russell, for her inspired suggestions and sage advice. Thank you all for your expertise and generous support and encouragement.

1

He told me I scattered sunshine everywhere I went and when I got old and wrinkly, my smile would never change. He used to send flowers to me at work, just because. One day he scribbled words onto tiny cream-colored cards that folded over to the size of postage stamps. One word per card. He popped them in secret places for me to find: my wallet, my running shoes, my undies drawer.

When I gathered them together and shuffled them around, his puzzle of words fell easily into place.

Hey beautiful—I love you

From a nice man.

2

For a long while after Dominic's death I thumbed back through time and tried to work out when it had all started, hoping to see through the blindness that had protected us during the early days.

A year or so after he died, my son Nic and I were driving home from the supermarket. Nic opened the passenger seat window without adjusting the air conditioning, just like his dad had done so often. It didn't matter how hot the day, he liked to feel the outside air brush over his skin. I switched off the air conditioner. Nic peeled off his T-shirt and threw it casually over his shoulder onto the backseat. I really needed a seat cover: stains of spilled food and mud from various soccer fields and dog paws were now integrated into the fabric design. He leaned forward, scavenging through the favored shopping bags he had placed at his feet. He opened a tub of Anzac biscuits we had bought on special. When were my two teenage sons not eating?

I pulled up behind a line of cars and waited at a red traffic light, next to a bus shelter housing a lone teenage Goth with one head-phone dangling from his ear. His long skinny legs, wrapped tightly in black denim, were stretched out along the bench and he was texting on his phone with two thumbs, faster than I can type.

"How do you tell the difference between Goths and emus?"

"Emo, Mom; for emotional."

"Right. Emo."

"You mean that guy?" Nic pointed to the boy at the bus stop. "I reckon he's emo."

"How come?"

"His jeans are tight and his hair falls down sideways over his face," he said. "Dunno. Goths push the dress-code thing a bit more. You know, trench coats, more chains and upside-down crosses and things."

He reached for another biscuit. "Can you drop me and Mitcho off at the movies tonight? Please?"

The emo in the bus shelter leaned back against a panel advertising Paddle Pops. *Delicious fun for the whole family to enjoy...*or something like that. Dominic had always been so fit and diligently health-conscious that it had seemed out of character when he started to devour whole boxes of Paddle Pops at a time. They had to be the banana ones. I didn't take too much notice at first. I laughed it off as an eccentric quirk and, on his fortieth birthday, the boys and I created an elaborate treasure hunt for him with rhyming clues. Buoyed by excitement, they didn't wait for him to decipher each one. They eagerly led him, clue by clue, through every inch of the house before the final clue directed him to the freezer in the kitchen and he found forty banana Paddle Pops awaiting him.

When did this quirky behavior move beyond endearing? Was it the day he made ten repeat trips to the same convenience store at the Mobil petrol station up the road, buying one banana Paddle Pop at a time? It was hard to know. The various whims slipped silently into a general continuum of puzzlement.

"You have *got* to be kidding," I had said at the time. "You're going back to get another one?"

"Yeah."

"Where's the impulse control? This is not like you."

He turned from me and, somewhat mechanically, made his way out the front door to get Paddle Pop number eleven.

"The light's green," said Nic, opening up the fresh orange juice and taking a slug. The humidity wafted into the car and joined my Paddle Pop thoughts as the idling engine and Nic's chatter about his best friend and the movie rumbled on. His voice floated over my ruminations that tried to make sense of things, that looked for the missing beginning to a story with a well-known ending. Some way to join the dots of realizations and say, *this is where it all started.* Wondering at what point I must have known that, while change had no identifiable beginning, change had already come. I pointed to the bus shelter before pulling off.

"I wonder how much of the Paddle Pop thing was illness?"

"You have to stop doing this, Mom. You'll end up writing off his whole freakin' life!"

Slapped by the wisdom flung at me, I moved on with the traffic.

We drove home in silence, his insight having hit the bull's-eye before I felt the sting.

By the time we turned into our street, the trees that lined both sides of the road had thrown up a canopy of leafy shade to welcome us home.

I waved at the neighbor over the hum of his lawnmower and pulled into our driveway, where we were greeted by two tail-wagging dogs. They never ceased to be excited by the sight of us, and their welcoming barks set off a chorus of yapping from the neighboring dogs over our back fence. Our home was nestled among a cluster of simple, low-set brick houses at the bottom of a hill. We were tucked in beneath the more majestic replica Queenslanders, raised high off the ground on stumps, with expansive, sheltered verandahs that seemed to float above the hilltop greenery. Nic picked up the bags at his feet and hopped out of the car. He opened the boot and gathered up the remaining shopping bags, ignoring the oranges that had rolled out during the drive home.

"Load me up," he said, holding as many bags as possible to save himself a second trip out to the car. Bags dangled off both arms as he opened his left hand for me to add the last two.

"You're already overloaded," I said, collecting the oranges.

"C'mon, I'm massive. Just do it!" I obliged his tease, and he grunted his way into the kitchen, Tarzan-style, before dropping the bags on the floor and rubbing the red lines that remained, crisscrossing their way up his forearms. I put the kettle on.

"Tea?"

"Nah." Nic took an apple from the fruit bowl and went through to the laundry. He stepped over a pile of sweaty sports gear and filled the washing machine one-handed while continuing to feed himself with the other. I unpacked all the cold items into the fridge and reached over to lift our now whistling kettle off the stove. I filled my mug with freshly boiled water and sat for a while at the kitchen bench, watching the tea stains drift from the tea bag in curious motions as the steam swirled.

A sudden mad scramble interrupted the peace as the dogs raced each other to the front door to welcome Michael home from uni.

"Hey!"

"Hey!"

Michael dropped his backpack among the grocery bags on the kitchen floor and leaned over to give me a kiss.

"Yesss! You've done a shop. What's there to eat?"

He went straight to the fridge, opened the door, and scanned the shelves filled with yogurt, milk, cheese, carrots, bok choy, broccoli, other leafy greens, and an array of fresh fruit.

"Mum?" He calls me mum, unlike his younger brother, who still uses the Canadian "mom." "Did you get any Tim Tams?"

"Nope."

"There's never any food in the house!"

The fridge door remained open as he waited for junk food to step forward. I reached in under him, grabbed two dog bones, and went outside. The dogs bounded out after me. Jessie, our Ridgeback cross, sat drooling at my feet. She waited obediently, long sticky globs of saliva dangling from her mouth, undistracted by Maxi, who pranced around like a wind-up toy and squealed uncontrollably in excitement. Maxi, our little black Kelpie, found it near impossible to "sit" and "stay" before receiving her treat.

Dominic adored dogs, and had spent patient hours training Maxi and Jessie. They were among the many reasons he had loved living in Brisbane: his dogs and the weather. He could be outside here—it was in the sunshine that his body and soul seemed most connected. We had moved to Australia from Vancouver when the boys were ten and eleven years old. His new position at the university here meant less travel than in his previous job, and he could spend more time at home. We got the pups within six months of arriving. Jessie was always the star pupil. She responded to all his commands, unlike anxious Maxi, who Dominic had despaired might never get the hang of it. He was a real dog man.

I remember the first time I went over to his house. I was still a teenager, a young girl in love with a young boy. His Doberman jumped up against the gate at the sight of me and barked viciously, shredding the air with her bared fangs. There was no tail-wagging and happy panting from this dog. My heart lurched into my throat. Dom took my hand.

"It's okay." His smile rested on me.

"Your psychotic dog is about to eat me."

"She knows."

"She knows what?"

His eyes brightened.

"You're just going to have to get over it," he said to the snarling dog. "Marie is here to stay."

The dog skulked away and sat with her back to Dom, refusing to look at him for the rest of the day. It had always been the two of them: playing fetch, going for runs together in the bushland that backed up to their home, sleeping at Dom's feet while he stroked her with his toes. She featured in important photos, too—he called her with his friendly whistle, and snaps were taken of them sitting together next to his newly awarded school sports trophies. Now there was me.

I smiled at the memory. The touch of Dom's hand and those soft blue eyes filled with wild tenderness when he looked into me. I watched Maxi and Jessie and, for a moment, I felt him again. I left both dogs gnawing their bones under the shade of a tree and came inside to wash their slobber off my hands.

I unpacked the remaining groceries. Cans on the second shelf, cereal on the third where the big boxes could fit, and washing machine detergent in the laundry. Not long ago, there had been no easy way to organize our life. Our world was out of whack. No matter how much we adjusted things, nothing seemed to fit.

Nothing much had made sense back then, least of all my dreams. Such vivid dreams that stayed with me, lodging themselves into the day. Dominic stood in front of me, encased in a gigantic ice cube. The ice was impenetrable. Hundreds of tiny cracks stretched their gnarled, splintered hands toward him. I tried to talk to him, but the sounds he heard were muffled by the thickness of the walls, and he couldn't understand what I said. So he watched the shape of me from inside his cell. He didn't seem to mind being there, but he was unreachable and the ice was making him cold.

Michael opened the freezer and added a handful of ice cubes to a beer mug of orange juice he had poured.

"Hey, Nic, wanna play chess?" he yelled across the house.

"Go to him, Mike, don't yell," I shouted from the laundry.

"Yeah," shouted Nic from his room, "but I'm going to a movie with Mitch later, so wanna play now?"

Dominic had taught both Mike and Nic to play chess when they were very young. They must have been about five and six years old. He could transform two wild animal children into calm little angels over a game of chess. Temporarily, anyway. We were living in Vancouver at the time and often took them down to Ambleside Park on the North Shore. It was a large beachside park with a view of Lions Gate Bridge hanging in the background, sprawling green lawns when they weren't bogged down from the rain, children's playgrounds, a dog park for four-legged friends, and the seawall that snaked its way along the water's edge where I loved to go running. A group of chess players would meet at the park regularly to play. One day, two older men sat across from each other at a portable chess table. Their coffees sat beside them on a low brick garden wall, untouched and growing cold. Nic's little blond head leaned in as close as he could to get a good look. The man wearing a black felt fedora looked up at Dominic, with a much shyer Michael sitting up on his shoulders, and smiled.

"Checkmate!" he cried out in a thick Polish accent.

"You want to play me?" he asked Nic. Nic looked back at Dominic, who nodded encouragement.

"I think this little man might beat you," said the loser of the game to his winning opponent. He ran both his hands over a full head of white hair and rested them on a very large belly.

"Can I watch?" he said to Nic.

Nic nodded and sat down on the brick wall. The man in the black hat rearranged the pieces to start a new game and positioned the board between them. He made the opening move and the game began.

Later that afternoon, a very excited little Michael bounced through the front door of our house, like Tigger, calling out the same thing we had heard throughout our car ride home. "Nic won! He won! Dad, I wanna play you. I wanna play you now!" Out came the chessboard, along with calm. They sat together by the fireplace, sliding chess pieces across the squares and munching on carrot sticks dipped in peanut butter. Dom stretched out on the floor, at the same level as Michael, and worked his usual magic. After some silent pondering and more carrot crunching, Michael took Dom's knight, feeling he had come up with this brilliant move all by himself. That day, Michael won, too. But the boys didn't always win. Losing offered all sorts of lessons, many of which ended in affectionate wrestles and squeals of laughter as their bodies tumbled together on the living room floor.

Chess games and lively affection for Dad went on for years, until Michael set up the beautiful wooden chess set we had given Dominic for his forty-first birthday. It was one of Brisbane's typical winter days—glorious sunshine followed by a cooler evening. It was still warm enough to eat ice cream, although we didn't have Paddle Pops this birthday. They sat across from each other, teenage Mike searching for the warm, familiar bond. Dominic stared ahead, disinterested.

"Dad?"

Dominic put his finger over a few pawns without moving them.

"Don't go easy; let me beat you properly," said Mike.

Dominic shifted in his seat, expressionless. "I don't feel like playing," he said in a flat monotone. He got up without looking at Michael and walked away.

Dominic started walking away from other things, too, like not turning up to Nic's parent-teacher meeting one evening. We had deliberately picked an afterwork time slot.

"Where is he?" asked Nic.

"He must be caught in traffic or something."

He didn't turn up at all. It wasn't the first time he'd done this. When we got home, he was watching TV.

"Where were you?" I said when the boys were out of earshot.

"At work."

"Is everything okay? Why didn't you call?"

"I'm the only one who can do the work."

"You missed Nic's parent-teacher interview."

He shrugged his shoulders.

"Dominic…?"

He looked at the TV.

"What's going on?"

"Nothing."

"Just when did these things become unimportant? There was a time you would have done anything for your kids…"

I was met with a blank stare and no reply.

"Dom, talk to me, please. Don't shut me out."

"I told you. I'm fine," he said.

He got up, walked away, and went to bed.

"What is *wrong* with you?!"

The boys' school activities had always been something we enjoyed together as a family, be they school plays, soccer or basketball games, karate tournaments—even torturous out-of-tune recorder playing. We went to parent-teacher interviews together, signed up for classroom reading, joined in on field trips, and were both on the traffic-duty roster. When Dominic was on lunch duty at their primary school in Vancouver, he played soccer with all the kids. The word was out: *He's so cool!*

He didn't go on about picking up litter; there was no need. The field would be clear of lunch wrappers on "Dominic days." Any litter went straight into the bin—the kids were ready and eager for a game. Mike and Nic had a "cool" dad. And, rumor had it, this tall, blue-eyed, and rather humble dad who cared about kids did not escape the attention of the many moms who seemed to hang around the school grounds just that little bit longer when he was there.

3

It takes time to settle into a new country. Moving to Australia was not our first international move, so we were familiar with the ups and downs of assimilating into a new culture and with the time it can take to feel you belong in a community. Looking back, I can see that Dom wasn't getting the same response from people here as he had in Vancouver. He was liked, but he wasn't engaging in the same way. He seemed more distant, and he was working harder. At the time, I thought maybe his new job was getting to him. The workload was enormous, but his colleagues were under the same pressure. We had talked about it with a couple of them one night over dinner. Good wine and wit infused the evening chatter, and the conversation expanded my sense of the departmental demands. The nature of academia seemed to be changing, and clearly they were all in the same boat. As time crept forward, the laid-back Dom, who absorbed life into his soul by playing in the sunshine, seemed more and more stressed.

One of my friends from work was throwing an Oktoberfest party.

I worked with great people and knew he would like them. Perhaps it would be good to get him out. Dominic's leg was bothering him, so I drove that night. He had been falling. His leg would collapse without warning, suddenly folding up under him like a puppet with a cut string.

"You really need to get this checked out," I said.

"It's just my gammy leg," he countered.

"But it shouldn't drop out from under you like that."

"It's nothing, really."

Dominic shrugged it off and stubbornly refused to see a doctor.

He attributed his leg's weakness to a car accident we had all been in many years ago, before we left South Africa. We were in our twenties back then. Nic and Mike were only eight months and two years old. The boys and I had a few cuts and bruises, but Dom sustained severe injuries. Had it not been for an off-duty ambulance that happened to drive by, Dominic would not have survived.

After extensive surgeries and several months in hospital, he was discharged to months more of daily home nursing. He was told he would never walk on it again. Against all odds and through sheer grit and determination, he was able to discard the wheelchair and then the crutches, and slowly walk back into his life. Acutely aware of being alive, he never complained. He had lived with chronic pain since the accident.

He learned to disconnect from it, determined to actively engage with his children. He had seen his life flash before him: a holographic review in vivid detail. He had clung on and now that he was back, his connection to family had intensified. Pain did not deter him. Along with chess games with the boys, he had fun bouncing them on the trampoline, riding a bike alongside them when they went for runs, kicking a ball around on the soccer field, and tobogganing with them because he couldn't ski. We did other things, too, like swim and kayak, things that were gentler on his damaged leg. And despite the pain, he joined me on forest walks, because he knew I loved being in the woods, in natural terrain, both tender and rough, where life felt precious and sweet. He felt it, too, he said.

All these years later, he paid little attention to his collapsing leg.

He dismissed the fact that it happened to his other leg, too, as well as my observation that he was becoming increasingly clumsy, frequently bumping into furniture and doorways as if he were unable to estimate his body's distance from things.

My friend who was giving the party lived quite a drive from us, on the other side of town. A few other colleagues would be there too. We worked together at an acquired brain injury unit—a neuropsychologist, a speech pathologist, an occupational therapist, the nurse unit manager, and me, the social worker. We were a good little team, and great friends. This would be the first time we would be meeting each other's partners.

Dominic and I stopped along the way to pick up a bottle of wine and some German pilsner to take along with our dessert. When I tried to pay, our debit card was declined.

That's weird. I know there's money in there.

"Try again, sometimes it's just the machine," said the cashier.

I tried again.

"Sorry, it's done it again," she said. "Says insufficient funds."

"Do you have any cash on you?" I said to Dominic.

He shrugged. I paid with the credit card and made a mental note to call the bank. It must be a mistake.

"Didn't you withdraw cash this morning?" I asked as we walked back to the car.

"Yes, sixty dollars. I had to get carrots."

"Hey, thanks. Did you get milk and bread? I was at Nic's soccer practice and never made it to the store."

"No, I had to get carrots."

"You spent sixty bucks on carrots?!"

"Well, I had to get carrots."

We drove toward the party, our conversation declining into another argument about money. There seemed to be less and less of it. It didn't make sense. Dominic did not seem bothered by it, but we were struggling to pay things like school fees when there should have been enough money in the bank. And anyway, why would we need sixty dollars' worth of carrots? We didn't even have a juicer.

"I needed carrots."

"You keep repeating yourself."

"That's because nobody is listening," he said.

We arrived at my friend's house. I shed the argument, applied my smile, and walked with Dominic into a party that was already well under way. My friend welcomed us at the front door wearing her naturally contagious smile, a lace-up-style dirndl dress, and a blonde wig covering her rich chocolate-brown hair.

"*Guten abend*, gorgeous!" She laughed vivaciously, giving me a hug and a kiss. "Hi, Dominic. I'm so pleased to finally meet you!"

Dominic nodded.

"Did you find us okay?" she said to him.

"No problem."

It was a bigger party than I had expected. The dining room table was laden with food. Warm potato salad, sauerkraut, and Black Forest cake sat among an assortment of other delicious-looking dishes. We made our way through groups of people wearing an array of colorful suspenders clipped onto rolled-up cargo pants, Bavarian aprons, and all-out lederhosen, and placed our *apfelkuchen* among the growing spread. The smell of barbecuing sausages wafted in from the deck. We grabbed a beer and made our way across the room to join some friends chatting to my boss. Our smiling host joined us and introduced her partner.

"So, what do you guys do when you're not at work?" he asked.

Dominic and I weren't doing half the things we used to do. When did Dominic last kayak? When was the last time we had people over? When did we last go for a bush walk, have a beach day, or go to a movie? I hadn't seen father-son chess games for over a year. Was it that long ago that he'd walked away from his birthday chessboard? We had stopped doing a lot of things we loved to do. What about the book we were going to write on our family history? When did we stop collecting those stories? Come to think of it, when was the last time we even discussed a good book? And *what* was going on when I came back from that great conference a few weeks before and tried to share my enthusiasm with Dominic over the new ideas I'd learned? I was used to his genuine interest in my projects, but he looked bored stiff. His only contribution was, "That's bizarre." He had repeated this remark a few times, until the flame those new ideas had kindled was extinguished.

"I hear you are a keen kayaker," my friend said to Dominic as she adjusted her blonde wig.

"I did it a lot in Vancouver. I haven't been out much in Brisbane."

He went on to describe some of the kayaking he and his best friend, Brian, had done in glacial waters north of Vancouver.

"You should come out with us sometime, we'd love you to join us!"

"That would be great," he said.

A jovial neighbor joined the group and interrupted the beginning of a conversation about preferences for river or sea kayaking. "So, Johnny's still our prime minister!" News was just out—John Howard had won the federal election.

"It's disgusting," Dominic blurted. "He's a damn fascist!" He swung his open hand to his head, not noticing the pause in the group.

People laughed somewhat awkwardly before they started chatting about the role of the media in influencing the electorate and what giving Howard a fourth prime ministerial term might say about the Australian nation in current times.

"It's an outrage!" Dominic interrupted. "He's importing political strategy from the US and fueling racial prejudice!"

The comments themselves were reasonable, but his intensity was bewildering. I squeezed his hand. *No, Dominic, not here, please, not here*, I willed him. He removed his hand from mine and walked off.

The TV in the living room was airing an election news story. Dominic went over to watch it. He sat on the couch but couldn't keep still. He stood up, sat down, and stood up again, shifting his weight from one leg to the other, sighing in protest. He frowned. Was he concentrating, or cross? My boss's partner was watching the TV and celebrating. She was pleased with the election result. Dominic turned his frowning face to her. "He's a fascist. He's a fuckin' fascist!"

Unlike the socially shy and retiring Dominic I had always known, this Dominic was unwavering in his argument. His usual social graces abandoned him, and he wouldn't let it go.

"This country is full of racists," he spat at her. "How else did he and his cronies get voted in with an absolute majority in the Senate?"

I cringed at how rude and emotionally volatile he seemed. This was so unlike him. He had lost custody of his tongue with, of all people, my boss's partner. How could I extricate him from this heightened conversation without causing more of a scene?

"Ze food is being served, *kommen und essen*, everyone, *ja!*" called out a friendly voice in an exaggerated German accent. The sausages that had been barbecuing out on the deck were ready. My boss put her arm around my shoulder. "It's okay, they can sort it out themselves, don't worry."

I welcomed the food interruption, but it was to no avail. Dominic stood in the crowd, folded his arms across his chest like a little boy throwing a silent tantrum, and flatly refused to eat a thing.

We left the party early. I drove home fuming. How would I face work on Monday? What would my colleagues think?

"Just *who* are you and where is Dominic?"

"What are you talking about? I'm Dominic."

"This is no time to be smart," I snapped.

I drove home in silence. Home toward the boys, with a stranger in the car. A stranger that was changing the shape of us.

For Mike and Nic, their dad had stepped over to the other side of the moon, and their mum was stressed out. Children of any age feel safe when their environment is predictable and nurturing, and they can trust the people within it, but as our life tumbled over, we thought Dominic didn't care about us anymore. As inconceivable as it was, he didn't seem to give a toss.

The boys no longer heard the friendly or affirming comments they were used to from their dad. It was impossible to understand what was unfolding and there was no way to take the guessing out of what might happen. How could I protect them? Was I adding to it all? Being a mother of teenage sons in turbulent times like this had me questioning if I knew what I was doing. I am under no illusion: there would have been times, even if Dominic had been more himself, that the boys would have let me know what a totally uncool mother I was. Michael might still have complained that he must have been switched at birth, landing with us by mistake, because we didn't understand him at all, and any real parents would. But it was hard to know what bits of these stormy moods were the result of our fraying family life.

"Calm down. What's going on?" I asked, joining Dominic at the kitchen counter when Michael came storming through like a fireball one night. In one long, tempestuous breath, Mike let me know that I didn't have a clue about what it was like for him to live in this family. And, and, anyway, who was I to tell him what to do? I couldn't make him do anything.

Dominic looked at Mike with vague disinterest.

"Could the alien that has abducted my son please return him to me unharmed?" I said. "I really miss him and would like to talk with him."

Michael's scowl did not veil his distress. He looked at me and then turned to Dominic. "That's just slack, Dad. Even I know that what I'm doing is wrong. You just stand there, when you should be supporting Mum. What's *wrong* with you?"

Shoulders slouched, he walked away, slammed the door of his room, and turned his music up, drowning us out.

Dominic stood at the kitchen counter, eyes vacant, face expressionless.

You used to be so reliable. Can't you see what's happening? The boys need you. This is supposed to be a partnership. Where the hell have you gone?

Dominic turned around and went to bed. I knocked gently on Michael's door.

I worried as I watched Mike and Nic try, in a variety of ways, to bring Dominic back, only to struggle with themselves when nothing they did had any impact. This was not their responsibility, but they wouldn't give up on him. They were kind; they did the eggshell walk; they challenged him; they completely lost their cool; and they pleaded with him to get help, just as I had done. The response was always the same: What were they on about? He was fine. He didn't need help. We were all bullying him.

There had never been any doubt before about family being Dominic's first priority, but there was no getting through to him now. I loved this man unreservedly; however, a fine line was developing between giving of myself and giving up myself.

"It's all so confusing. I don't know what bit I'm not getting," I said during a phone call to my brother, Patrick, in Los Angeles. My warm-hearted man was changing and I didn't know why. I kept churning the questions around in my head as if the mental agitation would help spew out an answer, but all I ended up with was a headache. I longed for my family, who had settled in America. We hadn't been in Australia long enough to share interconnected histories with our new Aussie friends. My rocks were overseas and the ground here was turning to quicksand.

I don't know when it all began. I no longer look for Paddle Pop beginnings or try to find order in confusion. But I can see how, over time, I made adjustments for Dominic as he changed—overcompensating, taking up the extra slack, finding all sorts of reasons to rationalize his changes in behavior. What started off as subtle and confusing became big and scary, and then I wondered how on earth it had snuck up on me. Before I knew it, I'd fallen down the rabbit hole and joined Alice in Wonderland. When I landed, I was sure I heard the Caterpillar ask, "Who are YOU?"

I didn't know. I just knew we were all different from who we had been before. So many things were changing. I kept asking myself what was real and what was not.

"I can't explain *myself*, I'm afraid, sir," said Alice on my behalf, "because I'm not myself, you see."

4

A mound of hard towels, fresh off the clothesline, lay stiffly on our bed, smelling of sunshine and waiting to be stroked back to their softer form. I stood at the foot of the bed, given over to the monotonous task of folding. Michael was in the study working on a school assignment. Nic was outside playing with the dogs. My gut shouted a warning.

"Dominic?" He had been with me a moment ago.

No answer.

A sudden stab of alarm awoke a protective instinct, a nameless knowing resting just below the surface. I dropped a worn beach towel, half folded in my arms, and hurtled down the hallway into the study to find Michael recoiling backward under Dominic.

"Let him go! Get your hands off him!" I shouted.

Michael was quiet and very still, trying not to inflame the situation. His frightened eyes wore the shaken look of someone who had seen a ghost.

"Dad, it's me. It's me, Mike."

I threw my body between them. Roaring like a mother bear, I shoved Dominic off Michael. Attack? From a man whose touch was gentle, whose affectionate hands had loved and held? I remembered how easily the boys would curl up next to him on the couch to watch a movie, even after a firm word. He had been an ass lately, but he had *never, ever* done anything like this before.

Dominic stumbled backward, raised his hands in relieved surrender, and said nothing. A look of confused horror crossed his face as he leaned against the three-drawer filing cabinet on the other side of the room, absorbing what he had done. Dominic's eyes had been dead for months, but that day I saw fear leap across his face and fill his eyes with panic so vivid that the image is permanently tattooed on my memory. Something was terribly wrong. Reactive, untamed, and disconnected—this was so unlike Dominic. He turned away and walked to our bedroom without saying a word.

I put my arms around Michael. "Are you okay?"

Stupid question—how could he be okay?

He nodded.

"Are you hurt?" I looked gently for marks.

He shook his head.

"What happened?"

"I don't know. It was so sudden."

Nicolas stood in the doorway looking smaller than usual. "I came as quickly as I could. Dad's so big. I didn't know what to do."

When the boys were as settled as they could be, I walked down the hall, past the photo wall bursting with happiness from another time, and into our bedroom. Dominic lay next to the towels on our bed. I stood facing him, my fury bubbling but contained, and delivered a calm but unequivocal ultimatum. "Get help, or we separate."

Dominic nodded without battle.

"In the meantime, I think you should go and stay somewhere else."

"No!" His eyes widened in protest.

"Why?"

"I'm staying here."

"Do it for the boys, Dom. We need to be safe. This is their home; they shouldn't be the ones uprooted."

"I'm not going anywhere!"

"Then we are leaving."

I took the boys and stayed up the road with a friend. She knew there were problems, but I didn't tell her exactly what had happened that day.

I was too ashamed. Was my marriage falling apart? Was he depressed? Was he having a breakdown? Something was wrong. Yes, he had a stubborn streak, but where was my gentle man of the past?

"Are you going to make an appointment to see someone?" I asked the next day when I went back home to check on him.

"Can you call? You know who's good," he said, seemingly detached from the dread of the previous day. We would see more of this detachment, but it would be a while yet before we understood why.

I made an appointment. We had to wait two weeks for the first session.

I worried about the boys. This could never happen again. I called Simon, an old friend, for help. He had known Dominic at high school in South Africa. He was the one person here who knew Dominic from long ago. He and his wife, Molly, lived on a property running a landscape business, a couple of hours north of Brisbane, in the Sunshine Coast hinterland. Immediately after we ended our call, Simon got in his Land Rover and drove down to our place. He took Dom out to a local coffee shop. They were gone for most of the afternoon. When they came home, Dom was quiet and very tired. He went straight to bed. Simon sat with me on the patio, confused by what was unfolding. It was clear from their conversation that Dom did not like what was happening either, but this was not the Dom he knew. Simon's laid-back, unassuming, intelligent friend had seemed uncharacteristically disconnected. He was calm, but something felt odd. Simon couldn't pinpoint it.

Dominic remained calm. Disengaged and calm. Simon kept in touch, as did Ed, another friend I had contacted. Ed lived a ten-minute drive away and dropped by most days to see Dom. We moved back home, and soon after, the sessions started. Dom asked me to come with him. Five months after his antics at my friend's Oktoberfest party, he was finally going to get help.

We found parking right in front of the counseling center. Dominic was always lucky with parking. No matter where he was or how busy the place, a parking spot would magically appear, just where he wanted it. We walked up the wooden stairs onto a large verandah. Two parlor palms in hand-painted ceramic pots framed the doorway to the waiting room of this newly renovated Queenslander. I took a seat in a squeaky wicker chair next to the magazine rack. Dominic remained standing. A young woman sitting opposite us looked up from her magazine and quickly averted her eyes when I smiled.

The counselor invited us into a cozy room furnished with two comfortable chairs and a blue couch scattered with colorful cushions.

A fresh jug of water and disposable drinking cups sat on a heavy wooden coffee table, alongside the mandatory box of tissues and a wilting potted plant that had had enough of everyone's sad stories and needed to be outside in the sun.

What am I missing? I thought as I listened. Dominic repeated the same stories over and over as if he was stuck in a loop. The counselor listened patiently, trying, without much success, to get him back on track. He was pleasant and polite, but he was rigid and strange. And his jokes weren't funny. They were harmless enough, but they were odd. They were empty and flat, a bit like him. *Maybe it's just me. Maybe I'm stressed and imagining things.* But something seemed weird about this conversation, and the next one and the next one. I just didn't know what. And I was embarrassed. I so wanted her to know the man I knew before all this. The man I knew was still in there somewhere. The man I wanted back. I continued to see glimpses of him, and I pinned my hopes onto them, but he was becoming harder to reach. He was trapped in that ice cube, the one from my dreams, and I could not penetrate the frozen walls of his jail.

Several months passed and the confusion became more familiar. Our counseling finished up—the counselor moved overseas, and we decided not to continue with someone else. The sessions weren't much help anyway; they had simply provided a stage for the repeated performance of Dom's disconnection. Perhaps confusion enveloped us all, preventing us from seeing the clues. It would be another year or so before we would fully understand why this kind of help was never the answer in the first place. In the meantime, life continued and Dominic got ready to leave for Sri Lanka on a work trip.

"You got everything?" I asked. He was kneeling over his open suitcase on the floor, struggling to fit everything in. "You normally have this packing thing honed. Today you look like me! What's not working?"

Dominic had always been a more logical and organized person than I had. When it came to packing, he used a list and had a system that was ordered, quick, and easy. I don't have the aptitude for neat jigsaw packing. I chuck things in and then sit on the suitcase lid, hoping it will close.

I watched him tussle. *What am I missing?*

I helped Dominic with the last of his packing and dropped him off at Brisbane's international airport. I kissed him goodbye and drove home to what I hoped would be a peaceful ten days. What was I missing? Why was I uneasy? He hadn't left me an itinerary like he usually did, nor did I have the usual list of contact numbers. Dominic was dedicated to the projects he was working on in Sri Lanka, particularly in places devastated by the 2004 tsunami and still in the throes of civil war. A town planner and academic with interests spanning housing, poverty, and post-war reconstruction in developing countries, he had relationships with universities there and had done some wonderful work with the Red Cross. However, I did not trust his ability to navigate the political complexities of such a trip in his present state.

Stop being ridiculous. Just enjoy the lack of tension at home. He'll be fine.

I shoved my concerns aside, chastising myself for overreacting. After all, things were generally better. And then, a few days before he was due home, I received a couple of bizarre emails from him that left me with visions of him in Jaffna, facedown in a ditch, blown up by one of the estimated two million land mines displaced by the tsunami and still lying about.

On the day of his scheduled return, I drove to the airport to collect him as planned, but he didn't appear. I waited in the pickup zone until I was ushered on by airport security.

"This is a three-minute zone, ma'am."

I went around a few times. Still no sign of him.

See, Dominic, this is why you should have a mobile phone, I admonished silently. But for as long as I'd known him, he had never been a phone guy. He wasn't a phone chatter to anyone, and his calls to me had never been characterized by long and delicious flirtations either. It would take some time before I would connect his current refusal to carry a mobile phone with confusion about how to use one. I parked in the short-term parking lot and went into the terminal. The electronic board said his flight from Singapore had landed an hour ago.

"It can take more than an hour to get through customs on busy days," said an airport attendant when I asked a few questions.

I looked at the electronic board. A Qantas flight had just landed from Auckland, and Dominic's flight dropped down yet another notch. Another twenty minutes went by, and another. Surely it wouldn't take an hour and forty minutes to get through customs? I called home. No, he hadn't arrived at home in a cab. Tired passengers continued to bustle through the causeway from all sorts of destinations, their luggage labeled with Qantas baggage tags, Emirates tags, British Airways tags....I would wait for one more person. I hoped to see him walk through in his favorite faded jeans and a tired, smiling face, but a set of laughing Jetstar flight attendants dressed in bright orange came into the terminal, pulling their wheeled suitcases behind them and looking as fresh as if they hadn't traveled anywhere. I overheard their chatter as they made plans to meet up for drinks that evening in the Valley.

I couldn't find an open service counter for his airline and was eventually directed to an enquiries office one floor down. Two well-groomed women with perfect hair and makeup greeted me. One was tall and the other short.

I didn't know if Dominic had simply missed his flight home from Colombo, was stuck in Singapore, or if he was in Jaffna and in some kind of trouble. He could only get in and out of Jaffna via military plane or a Red Cross boat. He hadn't emailed or called like he usually did if there was a change of plan. Communication from Jaffna was almost impossible. Did that mean he was there? It was so unlike him not to be in contact. He always let me know what was happening.

"I'm sorry, ma'am, we can't tell you anything," said the short attendant when I asked if they could tell me if Dominic had been on the flight, "but let's call security to see if they can help."

An official-looking man came in. The short woman left us and walked into a back office. The tall attendant continued working at the counter, tapping away on her computer with her shiny red nails.

"You'll have to go to the police with this," said the security man, without asking any questions. He pushed out his chest and adjusted his belt beneath a bulging belly. "The police have to go through all sorts of official procedures before the airport is allowed to release any information to anyone."

The phone rang out from under the folds of his protruding stomach. He reached down and tried to release it from his belt.

The tall woman looked up at me from her computer. "I'm a mother and a wife," she said. "This must be very distressing for you."

Her expressive brown eyes beckoned me to wait until she had the chance to say more.

"Excuse me for a minute," said the security man as he stepped outside the room to take his call. She waited for the door to close.

"Quickly—and this didn't come from me—Dominic's booking has been cancelled and he has not been rebooked on any return flight from Colombo."

"Thank you, thank you," I said, the relief loosening the knot in my stomach. A cancellation was much better than a no-show. Dominic wouldn't have been able to cancel his flight if he was in some kind of trouble. The security man came back in. He apologized for the interruption and continuously adjusted the phone on his belt, which refused to fit in its pouch as it should.

I thanked him for his advice and left the office, turning to thank the tall attendant with a nod that would not give her away. I drove straight home and contacted the university travel agent who had arranged Dominic's trip. I explained the situation, and she said she would make some enquiries about the cancelled flight. In the meantime, I rummaged through old paperwork from previous trips and found the phone number of Dominic's driver in Colombo. He confirmed that Dominic had been to Jaffna and returned. He said he was at the hotel in Colombo, but the hotel had already informed me Dominic had checked out the night before. No one seemed to know where he was.

At the end of a protracted day, the travel agent called. "Good news! He's just been rebooked on a flight home tomorrow." She gave me the new flight details. I imagined her hanging up after the call and shaking her head. *She must think I'm such a drama queen. All this fuss; maybe I really am paranoid and delusional.*

Dominic didn't seem the slightest bit perplexed to see me at the airport on the "wrong" day. He got in the car and said nothing at all.

Somehow, my worry, now tamed by relief, did not transform into a volcanic eruption of fiery words. Maybe some part of me intuited the need for containment, and I casually asked him what had happened. Unfazed, he told me that when he was at the airport, he had offered his seat to another person who was waiting on standby.

"The poor guy really wanted to get home," Dominic said. "I didn't mind."

The ability to plan is automatic for most of us. We don't stop to think about the complexity involved in sequential tasks. Only later would I realize how difficult it must have been for Dominic to plan what to do once he'd given up his seat. For him, giving up his flight was as simple as politely standing up for someone on a bus.

"Why didn't you tell me—do you have any idea how worried I was?"

No answer.

"Dominic?"

"You know, the airline said they couldn't give me another ticket, and when I tried to sleep the night at the airport, security kicked me out."

"They kicked you out?"

"Yeah, they bloody well kicked me out."

Dominic told me he'd spent the night outside on a street bench.

5

I pulled into our driveway after work and checked the post box for mail, as is my usual habit, and then made my way inside. Dominic's bicycle wasn't in the usual place leaning against the pool fence. He was still at work.

He enjoyed his rides to and from campus, although his leg was hurting more often these days. The weather in Brisbane made for a pleasant ride. He didn't need all the cold weather gear he had wrapped himself in when he cycled in Vancouver—though the cold didn't stop him swimming an ocean marathon in our other life back there. The boys were about eight and nine years old at the time. I remember being bundled up in our coats under a cold gray sky, along with all the other spectators, and cheering him on from the beach logs on English Bay.

"You look like a seal," Michael had said, watching his dad pull on his black wetsuit, booties, and hood.

Dominic grinned. "Let's hope I swim like a seal!"

He smeared grease over the exposed skin on his face and bent down so the boys could join in, helping to make sure he hadn't missed a spot.

"Wish me luck!" He put on his gloves, gave me a greasy kiss, and high-fived Michael and Nicolas before joining all the other seals at the starting line.

The warmth from those cold days seemed long gone. I made myself a cup of tea. The house was unusually quiet. Michael and Nicolas were at school, and the dogs were snoozing on the pool deck. I sorted through the mail on the kitchen counter. Half of it was junk. A collection of offers for gutter cleaning, the latest supermarket specials, and enticements to buy houses from grinning real estate agents all went straight into the recycling bin. The rest were bills.

Money was increasingly tight. Dominic couldn't explain it, and he normally did all this stuff. I hated all the detail of financial admin and was happy to leave this task to him. He had always enjoyed it, besides which, he could do all sorts of complicated sums in a flash in his head whereas I still relied on my ten fingers.

I went through to Dominic's study. It was even more cluttered than usual, and paperwork spilled out like exposed secrets from a series of cardboard boxes under the desk. Through a veil of dread, I saw flashes of the scene in the movie *A Beautiful Mind* in which Alicia discovers the bedlam in her brilliant husband's office before his diagnosis of schizophrenia. This wasn't quite the same; there were no secretly coded pictures pinned all over the walls. Our chaos was trying to hide in multiple boxes stashed under a workbench that stretched across the room from one wall to the other. Not knowing where to start, I sifted through the disarray of crumpled scrap paper, unopened bills, receipts showing some bills paid twice, unpaid school fees, and overdue notices that Dominic had squashed into the boxes now overflowing and spilling their contents onto the floor. We'd only had one box under the bench before—a small collection box for scrap paper. That box now had all sorts of documents that needed saving from the shredder, including his birth certificate.

I picked up a glossy blue envelope holding expensive luxury holiday packages Dominic must have purchased, unused and now expired.

The sunny invitation to family relaxation in places other than this had been hidden under the mess now laid bare on the floor. I opened the filing cabinet drawers. Folders were out of order; some were missing or lying in boxes; there was loose paper everywhere. What was I looking at here? Dominic had always been the organized one. How many times had he laughed affectionately at my more haphazard and "creative" filing methods? He was the one who helped me do the books for my private practice in Vancouver. And when a friend was in need with some business decisions, it was level-headed Dom who was the key intellectual contributor to logically isolating the best way forward. As for holidays, we never had a lot of money, but Dom had set up the Excel spreadsheet that helped us save for our annual camping trips down the Oregon Coast. We found all sorts of ways to have family fun on the cheap.

I moved over to the computer and logged in to our bank account.

My heart flopped around my rib cage like a fish in a bucket. I scrolled through our bank statements. In amongst the chaos and cash advances that could not be accounted for, I noticed we were supporting virtually every charity in Australia with enormous, generous donations that were automatically billed to our credit cards every month. Very Dominic to support these causes, but our accounts were virtually empty. We couldn't pay our bills—phone, electricity, property taxes, car insurance....School fees were due soon; so was the mortgage.

I sat back in the chair, my mind swirling with questions and curious recollections of unexplained financial stress, which always seemed worse when he was away. Like the time I asked him about the extra flights he had purchased in Vietnam on our credit card when the university had already paid for these tickets.

"I missed a plane. The stupid plane was late. I had to buy another ticket," he had said.

And the time he did not book the correct number of nights at the hotel in which he was staying and was moved to a luxury suite for the last two nights, at our expense. He didn't usually stay in these kinds of places anyway. They just gave him a new room, he had said, but he wasn't a luxury kind of guy. He worked in informal settlements and slums. It was hard enough to reconcile five-star resorts with gleaming marble floors towering over poverty without staying in a lavish suite.

And what about the time I had asked him where his expense receipts were? We needed them for our tax returns.

"They don't have receipts in Vietnam. I can't get them," he had said.

"Of course they issue receipts. People do business there all the time."

"It's a different system over there. They have no receipts there."

"Well, then, where are your Sri Lankan expenses?"

"They don't have receipts there either."

"Dominic?"

"What."

"Are you having an affair?"

"Don't be ridiculous!"

"Are you?"

"Of course not."

"Then what's going on?"

"Nothing," he had said, looking utterly confused.

The sound of Dominic's bicycle brought me out of my memories, back to the chaotic study and overflowing boxes spewing out his untidy thoughts and our family distress. It no longer felt like home; we were buried under the mess. Life is complicated, we all have messy rooms, but this clutter was taking over.

I could see him from the study window. He leaned his bike against the pool fence, stripped off his shirt and shoes, and dived into the pool in his cycling shorts. He swam a few laps and then hung on the side of the pool, cooling off. Maxi bounded over and licked his face, wagging her tail wildly.

"Piss off," he said, and climbed out of the pool. Dominic came inside and walked through to the study, still drying himself with a towel.

"She was just kissing you hello."

"I'm going back to Vietnam next week," he said, ignoring my comment and showing no reaction to the exposed paperwork all over the floor.

"What? You are going away again? Why all the trips?"

"I'm the only one who can do the work."

"You never used to like this kind of travel—wasn't that half the reason you took this stupid job in Brisbane?"

My attempt at a rational conversation about work-life balance, grandiose illusions of believing oneself to be the only person who can do a job, irrational spending, and the fact we were in shit street and headed for financial disaster went nowhere. Underneath the worry, my heart ached as the current of hurt swelled.

"I'm leaving in a week."

"Give me your credit card for our joint account," I said.

"Why?"

"Just give it to me."

"No."

"I'll have to freeze it, Dominic. I'm serious. Neither of us can use it anymore; it's maxed."

I took the card from his wallet.

"Just increase the limit."

"Something is wrong, Dom, and it's affecting all of us. It's doing us in. Please, you need to see a doctor before you go anywhere."

"Don't be ridiculous. I don't need to see a doctor. I'm fine."

Dominic left for Hanoi the next week—one month after sleeping outside on a street bench in Sri Lanka. On the second day he was away, an unshakable feeling loitered in my stomach. It clawed at my resistance until it toppled into my bloodstream like spilled ink and filled every part of me. Something was wrong. I called him at his hotel—a low-key, friendly place in the Old Quarter.

"I don't have any money," he said.

"What do you mean—were your cards stolen?"

It turned out that a cab driver had taken him on a five-minute trip that should have cost a few dollars, but Dominic gave him all of his cash: hundreds of dollars, the whole lot.

"Some people have it really tough over here. He was such a nice guy. He has a big family to feed and he earns nothing," said Dominic.

He then went to an automated teller machine to get more money but after he punched in the wrong PINs, it swallowed both his debit and credit cards. Three attempts, and they were gone. With no cash and blocked cards, he was in Vietnam without a penny.

"There's an ANZ bank in Vietnam, isn't there?" I asked.

"Yes."

I walked him through a plan on the phone, baffled; he still did so many other things very well. His unaltered skills in some areas created a deceptive mask that covered the things he now struggled with. This was beyond being a scatty professor. Things were looking too scary for that. Clearly, the counseling hadn't worked. He needed a different kind of help altogether and he simply refused to see a doctor. I would have to talk to his GP myself.

6

I took time off work the next day and went to the school to meet with two of Mike and Nic's teachers: the head of house and the dean of studies. It was a busy time of year. We met in the dean's office. Her desk was crowded with towers of student papers. A blurry-eyed teenager with the morning hair of a troll knocked on the open office door and handed her an assignment. From the look on his face, he had done an all-nighter. She smiled, thanked him, and closed the door. The three of us sat at a round table away from her marking. She poured me a glass of water while we exchanged pleasantries. Where would I start...

"Is everything okay?" she asked.

Is it that obvious? Tears welled as I slowly unzipped the story, exposing our life. Something was wrong with Dominic. I didn't know what, but family life was imploding. I was working at a community health center closer to home now and had increased my hours there to manage the financial pressure, but we couldn't pay the school fees, and I was worried about the boys. I didn't know what the future held. Life was messy, and I was here because the boys needed extra support.

"I have to ask you a difficult question," she said. "Is there any violence?"

God, I'm a social worker; this shouldn't be happening to me. How did it get to this? What if they report me to the department of child safety?

A million worries buzzed inside my head like flies.

"Dominic is away in Vietnam right now. Everyone is okay, but when he is home his behavior can be unpredictable and intimidating. It's so completely unlike him."

Empathetic nods.

"I'm going from here to speak to his GP."

"Could he be depressed?"

"I think so. I don't know. It's not easy to get him to accept help."

"It can be hard for men. Do the boys know you are here and what you are discussing with us?"

"Yes."

It was a warm day, but I felt gripped by cold and started to shiver. These two people had heard things I had previously not aired in public. Out from the shadows: a perfect family gone wrong.

I was offered a spare jacket and slipped it on, but when I focused on the boys—after all, this was why I was here—I didn't need it. The image of their faces radiated warmth and banished the shadows. The teachers and I talked through support options for them, from the school counselor to identifying those with whom the boys could establish trusted relationships—significant teachers, school friends and their families. We looked at managing homework demands. They reassured me their doors would be open to us at any time. I was offered support with fees and an invitation for the boys to board. They could be away from the turmoil while I focused on getting Dominic help.

The problem was Dominic did not think he needed help, and it was unlikely our family would stay intact if he did not cooperate. I had already met with a solicitor about how to protect the family financially while I tried to get Dominic medical help; about keeping my family safe; and about a possible separation, if that's what it took. He needed help and I was running out of options. Nothing seemed to be working.

After the school meeting, I walked down the school driveway and sat on a bench in the sunshine overlooking the main oval, collecting my thoughts, taking a breath. A ride-on mower hummed on the far side of the field and the breeze brought with it the fragrance of freshly cut grass. A boy clutching a violin case covered in stickers dashed past me on his way to the music center. A wet patch of sweat made its way down the back of his untucked shirt while an untied shoelace whipped the path dangerously close to his other foot. I wondered whether he would make his lesson on time.

I looked at my watch. It was time for me to go, too. I made my way to the car and drove from the school to the medical practice. Dr. Liam was running late, but when he invited me into his room, he wore his usual friendly smile. Always attentive, this man never seemed flustered.

"What can I do for you today?"

I sat down on the chair next to a plastic container of kids' toys. He wasn't my GP.

"I'm not here for me," I said.

I knew he could not tell me anything about Dominic, but I told him my concerns. I told him all the changes I had noticed, that I didn't know if Dominic was clinically depressed or having a breakdown, or if he had developed a mental illness or had a frontal lobe brain tumor. Our once lovely Dominic was changing. His sentences got stuck in repetitive cycles. He couldn't plan things like before. Maybe he was stressed and his brain was discombobulated, but he was verbally disinhibited, emotionally disengaged, belligerent, and at times aggressive. He didn't seem to be able to regulate his emotions. He couldn't read social cues of other people and he was spending all our money. I might have to leave, but I wanted him plugged in to help. I continued to glimpse the man I once knew through the whirl of confusion. It brought out the advocate in me, but while I was trying to look after my family, the responsibility of uncovering this unknown thing was too big and scary to carry alone. I needed Dr. Liam's help. If I could get Dominic to come in, could we arrange a scan?

I left the surgery and stopped at the supermarket to stock up on groceries before picking up the boys from school. Despite eating, Michael was losing weight. I popped in to the chemist to get some vitamins and an immune booster tonic. I arrived at the school early and was able to park in one of the coveted shady spots. Soon after the school bell rang, a throng of hot, sweaty boys in gray and blue took over the sidewalk. Mike and Nic came through the gate together. They passed two older boys wrestling on the grass before they noticed my car.

"Hey, Nic!" yelled a mate over the crowd and threw him a basketball.

Nic dribbled it through the mob of boys, deftly keeping possession. "Cheers for the ball, fellas!" He got in the car with it.

"Oi!"

"Is it yours?" I said.

"Drive, drive!" He turned a mischievous face to me and grinned. "Check this out."

He wound down the window and feigned a throw at the car parked alongside us.

"Niiic!"

He laughed and lobbed a three-pointer back to the crowd.

"Hey, how come I always get the backseat?" said Mike as he got into the car.

"Payback for all the years you told me I would get arrested because it was illegal to sit in the front seat until I was twelve."

I started the ignition. "How was your day, guys?"

"Good," said Nic.

I looked at Mike in the rearview mirror.

"Yeah, good," he said.

"How was the meeting?" said Nic.

"They were very understanding."

"Like, what did they say?" asked Mike.

We talked about the meeting as I drove—how the teachers would now be able to understand some of the pressures they faced at home; that they wanted to know what each of them might need; that they acknowledged they might each need different things at different times; that they hoped the boys would feel comfortable to go to them; and that I would continue to be in regular contact with them.

"They also said you could board."

"No way, I'm not boarding," said Nic.

"Me neither," said Mike.

"It might be really good. I'd be close by. We'd see each other all the time. You could be weekly boarders."

"Everyone will think we're problem kids. That's who goes there, you know," said Nic.

"That's not so," I said.

"It is," said Mike. "At least for the boarders whose families live ten minutes from the school."

"You'd be able to play, to study and concentrate, and to know I was getting help for Dad."

"I don't want you at home alone with Dad," said Mike.

"Yeah," said Nic. "We'd just be worried all the time."

"At least if we're home, there are three of us," said Mike.

7

Dominic began to swing from calm to anxious and confused to unpredictable more often. He never raised a finger against anyone like he had that wild day in the study, but I never knew if he would. Dominic had come home from Vietnam, brushing off the money incident as if it never happened. The circles under his eyes were dark enough to look like smudged mascara. He was always tired and took more naps during the day. He said he was overloaded at work; he would probably look for a new job. Simon made the two-hour drive back to Brisbane again to check on his friend and to see how the boys and I were doing. He had tickets to a Springbok-Wallaby rugby test match and took the boys along for some fun.

I worried about Michael and Nicolas, and I watched them both worry about me. They were too young for this burden, and I didn't know how to relieve them of it. At the end of a day, as the sun slipped down over the horizon, it took with it some of Dominic's light. Increased agitation and confused pacing became more familiar in the shadow that fell before bedtime.

"Sundowning," they would eventually call it. What I didn't realize until much later was that the sun had in fact held on to what was precious, slipping over the edge of the world with the pieces of Dominic it had been able to save and returning them to him again after he had slept.

At the time, however, our hypervigilance switches were set to automatic and, when Dominic became agitated, the boys wouldn't leave me alone with him. If we got annoyed or told him to stop, it got worse. We started to walk around on eggshells, and, again, I felt sick at recognizing the signs of our adaptation to his behavior. How had I found myself in a situation of such domestic volatility? How could I protect the boys? As soon as I noticed signs of a shake-up, I took them out on drives to sidestep the storms.

"Let's go," was all I had to say.

They gathered their homework, or came as they were. No fuss— just a quick swoop and routine exodus. I can't count the amount of McDonalds sundaes we consumed during this time. Cheap snacks I could barely afford. We caught up with the day and the various homework assignments that did not require a computer. We didn't have a laptop to do homework on the run. I sat at those peach-colored tables drinking cheap coffee and wondered if these precious boys of mine would rather be outside in the parking lot, vandalizing walls with graffiti or smoking joints behind my back, escaping the world they found themselves in.

On one of these evening evacuations, Nic leaned forward in the front seat of the car. He put his elbows on his knees and cupped his head in his hands. He cried until he almost broke in two. I reached over to catch the sobs and hold his heaving back.

"I wish one of my friends would call me right now—just so they would know. I would pick up and be crying. They'd hear me, and they'd *know*," he said, words swirling around in tears.

"Would you like to call someone now?"

He shook his head.

"And like, I can't just go to school tomorrow and tell them stuff either," he said, lifting his head up to look at me. "I don't know what's going on with Dad. And even if I did, today would be over by then. It would just be words."

The remnants of the evening would be hard to capture; they would be scattered like feathers into the wind. He put his head back in his hands.

"It's hard to explain—they wouldn't really *know*. But, maybe, if someone phoned right now..."

"It wouldn't be so invisible?" I said.

He nodded.

Their world was crumbling. They didn't know how to talk about what they did not understand, and they were unable to control a life that had once felt safe and stable. Mostly, they grieved for the dad they knew and loved, and they worried about what our future held as a family. I reassured them none of this was their fault and that there was nothing they could do, or not do, to make their dad better, but I knew this didn't shield them from what was happening at home. What I did know was that this wasn't good for them, and I was going to have to make some decisions.

When we came back home from our drives and entered the familiar tentative air, Dominic had usually put himself to bed. It was as if the weather had settled but remained vaguely ominous. He would wake later with no sense of what had taken place. We didn't know which was worse: the agitation necessitating our flight from the house or his glaring indifference upon our return. And then pieces of him would return. There were periods of reprieve when he took an interest in homework and there was laughter and play—only to cycle inexplicably back into disconnection and confusion.

No matter how many times I asked him to, Dominic continued to refuse to see a doctor. How was I going to get him in there so he could be referred for a scan? Was he in denial? I searched his face for a secondary emotion—stubbornness, fear, something. There was nothing but a blank canvas.

Patrick called from Los Angeles to check in on his big sister. We talked through all the ins and outs of our crazy life—he has a great capacity to listen, my brother. He told me he would be coming out in a few weeks. He did this several times over the next couple of years.

"How are the boys?" he asked.

"Exams are coming up. Michael's got QCS in a few weeks."

"What's QCS?" The system in America was quite different.

"It's the statewide exam for all Year 12 students. The scores affect the ranks kids get to gain entry to university courses."

The night before Michael's QCS, the boys were in their bedrooms.

It was almost 9:30 p.m. Nic was getting ready to pack it in for the night, and Mike was sitting at his desk, working on the computer. Their doors faced each other. If they left them open, they could see and talk to each other from their beds. I heard their chatter from the kitchen. The house felt lighter. Dominic had been more like his former self over the past few days, and the sparkle of laughter had reentered our home. I was hopeful. He had even played water polo with the boys in our pool.

Without warning, a storm came tearing down the passage.

"Dominic?"

He strode past me.

Our house was small, too small to run indoors, especially for a man as tall and well built as Dominic. A photo frame smashed to the floor as he bumped into the wall in his frantic pacing, back and forth. The boys' rooms fell silent.

"Dominic!"

He accelerated, as if desperately trying to escape from some-where, frenetically pacing the same route—an invisible straight line along which he was being flung back and forth. A kitchen stool toppled with a clang. He startled at the noise and barged through Michael's bedroom door to get away, tripping onto the bed, using his arms to brace against his fall. He bounced up and swung around, leaving the room as fast as he had entered, continuing his dash to nowhere. Without noticing, he had accidentally scattered Mike's papers all over the floor.

"You have to get dressed for school," he said to Nic as he passed his door. "He has to get dressed for school," he said again to me, with increasing urgency. He did not enter Nic's room. He would have had to turn right and this storm did not allow him to change direction spontaneously.

His eyes were fixed, wide open, unblinking, but it was as though he couldn't see anything. He strode his commanding body back into the family room; back to the end of the line in Michael's room, through the papers on the floor; back to the family room—resolute pacing, back and forth.

"Dominic."

He didn't seem to hear me. His agitation was not directed. It was as if we weren't even there.

"Come!" I said to Mike.

I closed the door, locking the three of us in Nic's room, and sat on the floor with my back against the door. We sat in silence, listening. Dominic did not try to come in. Nic's room was off the pacing route. We heard the commotion move back and forth. I don't know how long we waited before the storm quieted, but when I heard a calmer Dominic in the kitchen, I slowly opened Nic's door. He was walking without bluster, and the fear in his face had gone.

"Dom?" I said his name calmly.

He looked at me as if I was someone he didn't know. I smiled, posing no challenge, hoping to contain things. He smiled back with the fresh innocence of a child.

"Come, you look tired. Would you like to lie down?" He followed me to our bedroom and put himself straight to bed. The boys hovered at our bedroom door.

"It's okay," I mouthed to them, but they stayed there.

Five minutes later, Dominic was asleep. Michael had a shower, and I made both boys cups of rooibos tea with honey. Nic helped Mike gather up the trampled papers on his floor in silence. They stacked them in a pile, trying to straighten the crumpled ones, but the creases were deep and looked like fresh scars. They climbed into bed, leaving their doors open so they could see each other. I sat on Mike's bed, leaning my back against the wall as they talked.

"Why won't Dad get help?" said Nic.

"I don't know, angel."

"I don't like it when he's away, but I don't like it when he's here either."

We sat together, absorbing life as we did not know it, until the mugs were empty and there was nothing more to say. I kissed them goodnight, wishing I could undo the evening. Then I took a look around the family room. I swept the floor and carefully removed the broken glass from the fallen photo frame. Dominic and the boys beamed back at me from the glassless photo with carefree smiles. I remembered the laughter and wrestling that had taken place on the lawn after this photo had been taken, when they were all dressed up in fancy clothes for a wedding—that and the white chocolate fountain surrounded by fresh fruit and other goodies the three of them had gorged on. I had chosen this sleek black frame five years before because of the large white cardboard insert that could be hand decorated. The boys' bright potato prints had not lost their color, although the yellow T and D in HAPPY FATHER'S DAY, printed in their handwriting, had faded.

Mike came through and stood in the doorway. His eyes were puffy from tears of liquid stress.

"I can't sleep," he said.

I went through to his room and held my distraught child in my arms, stroking his head until, utterly exhausted, he fell asleep in the late hours of the night.

Michael walked into his exam the next day with the night heavy on his shoulders.

The boys were again offered the opportunity to board at school, but they were both adamant about staying home with me. Dominic flatly refused to stay with anyone else, and he was clearly not safe on his own. Even if he was, we were flat broke. I had no way to afford the rent of another home or even a small apartment for the boys and me. Without a diagnosis or a treatment plan that could be enforced, I set up homes away from home for the boys with good friends where they could stay or go for mini-breaks. They were able to come and go as they needed and there were times when I insisted on it.

In the meantime, I put together a report that would accompany the school's support of special consideration for Michael's Year 12 exam results. As it turned out, we did not need to submit it. The year had been a blur for him and, disappearing into the fantasy land of complex strategy computer games instead of study, he found a simulated realm where he applied his ability to be creative, think strategically, apply economic theory, and, despite everything, come out on top and rule the world! One of his teachers wrote on his school report, "I'd like Mike to be my prime minister."

As the end of the year drew near we were no closer to knowing what we were dealing with. Life at home and school continued despite the ongoing wild rides on Dominic's emotional roller coaster.

When the head of house asked Nic to represent the Year 11s in farewelling the graduating Year 12s at a house assembly, he singled Mike out in his speech. He spoke about how proud he was to be Mike's brother, saying that Mike's support and care meant more to him than anyone could ever know. His speech was met with a choral *awww*, mockingly thrown up at him from the crowd of teenage boys. Joining the tease, Nic hammed it up, laughing as he caught his brother's eye.

Michael had had no idea this speech was coming. He replied with a reserved smile, quietly polishing his knuckles on his chest.

The hidden story would not have been known by all the boys there, but a couple of friends and the teachers were aware of the subtext. They had been through a tough year together. This was a public thank-you and an acknowledgment in front of a hundred and fifty boys that they would look out for each other.

8

I worried about something happening to Dominic overseas, yet simultaneously welcomed the peace in our home when he was gone. The boys were noticeably more relaxed when he was away.

Dominic had always been a genuinely modest man: his identity had never been wrapped up in work. This frenzied desire to travel so much didn't make any sense. What I did know was that Dominic's work had become a strange obsession—a significant departure for the quietly passionate, laid-back homebody who, right back to his first job out of university, had taken time out in his day to play soccer with kids in the South African townships where he worked. There was no doubt of his commitment and drive, fueled by a belief in social justice—we shared those values—but he had always invested in a life outside of work, and this was a man who knew how to play.

Dominic's brother Daniel wrote a series of reflections for the boys about his big brother, some of which reflected these ways of living.

> Talking about [Dominic and his work in] townships in South Africa reminds me of one story I always enjoy. There was a famous soccer player from South Africa in the 1970s and 1980s called Gary Bailey, who couldn't play international soccer for our country because of the sporting sanctions, and

so he took advantage of his British parentage. He ended up playing goalkeeper for Manchester United and England for many years and was famous in South Africa. Well, Dominic used to work in soccer-mad townships, and had more than a passing resemblance to Gary Bailey, so every time he was walking in the streets, the little kids would run around pointing at him saying, "Gary Bailey, Gary Bailey." Imagine what happened when he kicked a ball around with them.... Dominic always quite enjoyed the mistaken identity.

I had no idea if fantasy kicked a ball around with reality in the current game of our life. But life was changing. When we lived in South Africa, Dominic's work was on our doorstep and there was no travel. When we moved to North America, the nature of his work required regular travel, and it was the source of ongoing internal conflict for him, especially after three years as the home-based parent while he did his PhD.

"I want to be part of the kids' life. You know, the everyday stuff," he had said, feeling displaced by a job that took him away from home more than he liked. Some travel was fine, but not this much.

"You don't get that time back," he had said. "No job can entice me away from that."

Some people love constant global travel. He didn't. This had played a role in our move to Brisbane. He would have time with the family doing everyday stuff he missed. So what was he doing?

His next trip was to America and Canada. He was presenting at an international conference. This was the confusing part. There were things he still managed very well. I didn't see him in his work environment so I had no way to tell how things were going, but his paper had been accepted and he was still publishing. It seemed his students loved him. He received great evaluations from them and, given the work he said he was churning out, he appeared highly productive. I wondered if the problems were only happening at home. However, he did say he was looking for a new job because the bastards in the department didn't really understand him. He had arranged several meetings on this trip regarding academic positions back in Vancouver.

I love Vancouver. We have lifelong friends there and moving back would mean I would be close to my family. I missed them terribly—I'd go back in a flash—but a move now, like this?

"I'm not going anywhere until whatever is wrong has been sorted out. I'm not moving again just to take this monster back over there with us."

"What monster?"

"I mean it. I'm not moving."

"Well, then, I'll go alone," he said.

"This is insane. A move is not the solution."

Pause.

"Can't you see what's happening? Something's not right, Dom. You know it's not. Please, see Liam before you fly out."

"Don't be ridiculous."

Dr. Liam had already discussed our situation with a neurologist and a psychiatrist. They were waiting in the wings, ready to see Dominic as soon as he agreed to an appointment, but—despite my updates of unfolding anarchy—without any kind of medical assessment from anyone (not even his GP), things were still too gray to enforce any kind of medical evaluation. Dominic left without seeing a doctor, determined to sort out his future overseas.

Friends there noticed a change in Dominic. I wasn't imagining things. It was strangely validating, but confirmed my fears. At least if I had imagined it all, maybe overreacted a bit, we might be able to look back one day when the stress was over and remember it as a crazy, troubled time.

"He said the cab driver got lost," said Grace on the phone. Grace had known Dominic for as long as I had. She and I went to high school together in South Africa and had developed a bond that continues to nurture us through life. Dom and her husband, Graham, were good friends, too. They went back a way—they had been at the same high school in Durban, together with Simon. Our two families had ended up in Vancouver, our kids attending the same school and growing up together like cousins. Dominic was staying with them, in a neighborhood he knew like the back of his hand. He didn't turn up for dinner after a meeting at the university. Turns out he ended up in the wrong suburb and couldn't find his way home to them.

I heard from others how easily agitated he became, how he repeated himself so many times, how he said strange things. It wasn't like him, they said.

No one could put a finger on the exact problem, until Dom met with my sister Reagen in San Diego on his way home to Australia. She adored Dominic. She is eleven years younger than I am and had known him since she was eight years old. He had played with her as a little girl and, as she grew older, he was the one she turned to for all her boyfriend advice. She and Dom had planned to meet at a set time and place, but he didn't turn up. She called his best friend, Brian, with whom he was staying. Brian and his family had moved from Vancouver to the sunny shores of this Californian city shortly before we moved to Australia.

Yes, said Brian's wife. They had dropped him off at the mall; he should be there. Come to think of it, though, they had had a similar experience: Brian couldn't find Dom at the airport when he flew in. He had searched for ages and eventually found Dominic waiting patiently, with no sense of time, at the wrong terminal.

Reagen spent three hours looking for him in between calls to me in Australia and checking in with Brian's family in the event he had gone back to their place. Finally, she found him in a coffee shop somewhere.

After spending the afternoon with him, and chatting between his repetitive and inflated compliments about her earrings, she offered to drive him back to where he was staying. He declined, saying Brian would pick him up after his shift at the hospital where he worked as a doctor.

"His shift ends at midnight."

"I'll wait."

"But everything here will be closed up."

Reagen insisted on taking him home, but he couldn't tell her where Brian lived. She called them to get directions and drove him right to their front door. Dominic didn't recognize the house.

She called my dad in tears.

"What do I say to Marie?"

"Tell her everything. She's looking for input. Tell her everything."

The phone rang. I picked up. "Rea?"

She told me the details of the day with anguish. "He's not himself at all, sis. It's like he has Alzheimer's or something...."

Her words fell with a clang into my gut, reverberating there with my own intuitive dread.

The more stories I heard, the further the reverberations traveled, and when I learned what had happened when he went for a walk "to get away from things" during the conference at the beginning of this trip, every part of my body was on high alert. He got lost in an area most would not wander through alone, and said he was robbed by a gang of about eight young men, one of whom held a gun to his head.

I went to bed that night with a cracking headache, playing over in slow motion all the near-misses and potential upcoming catastrophes.

I had no idea what was real or not, but clearly, Dom was not safe. I went in to see Dr. Liam the next day, sharing every detail given to me by friends and family on these calls. I did not know Dominic's colleagues in Asia, so this was the first time I had been able to collect collateral history from people who spent time with him while he was away. A doctor's appointment was set up for him the day after he returned.

As Dominic unraveled, I learned to juggle my emotional responses with practical tasks, guided by what felt like a pair of over-active antennae on the top of my head registering all stimuli within a 360-degree radius. I said nothing of these overseas escapades to the boys, but I was tuned in and ultra-aware of the stress signals barraging my family. As I juggled the known with the unknown, I worried about what might happen if I dropped any balls.

We were losing Dominic. He had entered a strange and vague world, a kind of theme park filled with roller coaster rides and distorted mirrors; a kind of Wonderland except, unlike Alice, I didn't know if he would find a way back.

I drove to the airport to collect Dominic. I knew he was on the plane. Brian had driven him to Los Angeles and seen him off. He was tired from the long trip but unflustered. I said nothing of my worries. We made small talk. He hadn't slept much on the plane, he said.

"I was at the doctor the other day, and he said there are some new requirements for travel shots. He'd like to see you," I said as we drove home.

"Okay."

The next morning, I drove him to his appointment. He did not question the prescribed CT scan or the referral to a neuropsychologist for cognitive testing. Who goes in for travel shots and doesn't ask questions when he's told he needs a brain scan?

We went straight from Dr. Liam's rooms to the hospital with the referral.

Examination required: CT scan—brain
 Reason for investigation: Perseveration, behavioral distur-bance. Cognitive change?

The initial scan was inconclusive.

"You see," said Dominic when the results came through. "I told you, I'm fine."

There was no tumor, but something was stealing Dominic away and I didn't know what it was leaving behind. Despite the questions, we couldn't find answers. Our walk through Wonderland was getting wilder as nothingness was whipped up around us.

There was a three-week wait for an appointment with the neuro-psychologist for cognitive testing, and the earliest neurologist's appointment was after Christmas, in seven weeks' time. The Christmas closures were slowing everything down. Dominic agreed to see Dr. Liam in the meantime. After all, his scan was fine, and he would be off again soon. Yes, he was tired, and he needed a break, but so what if Dr. Liam had booked him off work for a month? It was very nice of him to do that, but he would take the break later. He was the only one who could do the work and he was all set to go on his next trip.

The week after the scan, we went to one of our follow-up appoint-ments with Dr. Liam. The air-conditioned waiting room provided welcome relief from the oppressive Brisbane humidity. Dominic flipped through a few magazines without reading them and started to jiggle his knees. A baby screamed from inside Dr. Liam's consult-ing room. Shortly thereafter, an exhausted-looking pregnant mother with a blotchy-faced toddler in her arms came through the door. Dr. Liam smiled as he said goodbye to the tearful child and then turned to Dominic.

"Hi, come on in," he said. Dominic returned the smile and went into his office.

At the same time, my GP, Dr. Kym, walked up the hallway to her room opposite Dr. Liam's.

"Hi!" she said. "Do you have a sec to pop in?" I followed her into her room and she closed the door. She said she'd seen me in the waiting room a few times with Dominic. Was everything okay? And why was I looking so tired and dreadfully skinny?

With the focus suddenly on me, I burst into tears. In one long, wet breath I blurted, "Dominic's-lost-his-marbles-I-think-he-has-dementia."

The D word. The thing I dreaded but had not dared to say in case it came true. The fingers of fear clawed at my stomach.

"I know it's *impossible* 'cause he's so young, but…"

"That's not like Dominic at all," she said after I talked some more and relayed a story about his pacing up and down, up and down, looking for himself and finding nothing. From the kitchen to the dining room and lounge, back to the kitchen, through to the dining room and lounge. She remembered the Dominic she had met soon after we had arrived in the country, the dad who brought his sons in when they had fevers or ear infections—how he sat with them as they flinched when their plantar warts were being zapped with liquid nitrogen. She remembered their affection; she remembered wishing there were more dads like him.

Just the evening before, Nic had been sitting on the kitchen counter as I prepared dinner, swinging his legs and leaving black scuff marks from his shoes on the cupboard doors beneath him. The repetition of Dom's pacing had started to fray his nerves.

"STOP! Aagh, Dad, please. Just stop!"

Dominic had swung around and grabbed Nic by the arm. I told Dr. Kym what had happened when Dominic felt the interruption of my firm hand on his. How his blue eyes had pleaded with me from behind the bars of his caged brain. How, without noticing Nic's ashen face, he had opened his fist, stood there frozen for a few seconds, and taken himself off to bed.

"I don't know what to do," I said. "He thinks there's nothing wrong. Dr. Liam's got him on sick leave, but he insists on traveling. He's unstoppable. He's not safe. I don't want to wait until something terrible happens before we act and do something."

I was sleep-deprived and too thin. She asked if I would come in to see her again.

"I'd like to be there for you, help make sure you are okay while Liam gets to the bottom of this with Dominic."

My check-ins with her gave me a view out of Wonderland and a forced break away from what soon became round-the-clock care. During the year to come I flooded her office with rivers of accumulated grief and carer exhaustion so overwhelming I could hardly stand straight. She witnessed our unfolding story, she listened, and she shared in the tears. She reminded me that I was "normal," and she encouraged me to write this book. I have encountered many medical people in my work life who have reduced their patients to a series of symptoms, entered into medical charts in unfamiliar language. Dr. Kym never overlaid our experience with a stamp of official scientific expertise; she listened beyond that and held my grief most tenderly. Together, she and Dr. Liam stepped in with tangible humanity and became an integral part of our strangely unfolding journey.

Two weeks before Christmas, a neuropsychologist came to our home to do an assessment and, on his advice, I took the boys out to minimize any distractions. It was school holidays. The Queen Street Mall was humming with the beat of live buskers, sporadically interrupted by the screeching laughter of teenagers who had gathered there to flirt with each other. The boys stopped off to get a Boost Juice.

"Check it out—two o'clock," said Mike.

"She's hot!"

"Smokin'!"

They slurped on their smoothies, and Michael stopped at the window of a hobby store to look at model airplanes.

"Hey, Mum, check out this model!" he said.

"Is it a Red Cross plane?" asked Nic.

"Ha ha," I said and walked over to have a look.

Mike had started making model airplanes when he was six or seven years old. Our kitchen table became an aeronautical engineering site from which planes and rockets would be launched into outer space, beyond gravitational pull, and then orbit the earth as they dangled from the boys' bedroom ceiling. Numerous aircraft would hit Dominic's head as he entered their room, setting them all off in yet another fantasy battle high in the sky. I usually reframed this as a peace and rescue mission, or a food and medical supply drop.

Back in those days, little Michael had had his eye on a new plane for a while and I had offered to take him to the store.

"I'll take him," Dominic had said as Mike ran off to get his coat.

"Why?"

"Because if he goes with you, the poor kid will come home with a Red Cross plane."

"What's wrong with a Red Cross plane?"

"He wants a WWII model."

"But…what about our thoughts on war toys? I thought we didn't want to encourage any ideas that suggest violence is the best way to settle disputes. C'mon, we both prefer toys that help the boys use their imagination to build and create, not to destroy."

"But there's a story to tell them here. This is about world history; there's lots to learn. Let's go get a warplane!"

The boys and I laughed at the memory and continued walking through the crowds doing their Christmas shopping in the outdoor mall.

"Yeah, we know," said Nic, giving me an affectionate nudge. "No guns and no objectifying women."

"Hey, check out that rack!"

"Hell yeah!"

"Out of 10…?"

"Oh, 8, maybe 8.5?"

They looked at me.

"Almost, almost…!"

I smiled.

"Nah—she's not taking the bait."

They both collapsed laughing.

9

It would take a week for "concerning" results to come back from the neuropsychologist and a while longer before we would fully understand the turbulent storyline of our current lives. More tests needed to be conducted. Dominic refused. He said he had "passed the test." What were we on about? He was fine. Of course he was off to China after Christmas.

Simon and Molly suggested we spend Christmas with them. We could stay a few days. It would give us a break, they said. On Christmas morning, I noticed Molly walk away from the Christmas tree, trying not to show her distress as she watched Dom's emotional disconnection swing to rigid reactivity. He paced relentlessly and ate with no self-regulation, and when he went for walks through the nurseries on this beautiful rural property, he said he saw massive snakes. He gesticulated, showing me the size of their girth with his hands. First there were five, then six, then eight. The number kept changing but the description stayed the same.

The visit made no difference. Dominic was supersensitive to perceived criticism. If Simon mentioned his observations or offered to support his friend in getting help, Dom insisted he was fine and became agitated. "It's like he has schizophrenia or something," said Simon.

Despite being on sick leave and under medical advice not to travel, a few days after we came back to Brisbane and only six weeks after being lost and held up in America, Dominic left for China. He didn't care about missing the neurologist's appointment that had been booked. According to Dominic, he didn't need to see him anyway. I frantically tried to get a medical injunction to prevent him from going. I didn't want him to hit rock bottom or have something awful happen before we could step in. Things were bad enough as they were, and he wasn't safe. But despite the risks, a diagnosis was still too inconclusive, and I was told there wasn't enough evidence to be able to intervene. Short of darting him with a sedative and chaining him, unconscious, to his bed, there was no stopping his travel.

"You're going again?" said Nicolas.

"You'd better not miss Mum's birthday. If you don't come home for her birthday..." said Michael.

If Dominic was retreating to something he knew so that he could escape the turmoil of his condition, it provided no relief. It simply traveled with him. In fact, things were always worse when he was away from home. While his teaching material was familiar, easily accessible from his long-term memory and relatively free from confusion, China was not. In a new environment, he was unable to plan or to navigate and his symptoms were significantly exacerbated. I will probably never really know what happened there, but for much of the time, I had no idea where he was or when he was coming home.

Initially, I had thought he wouldn't be able to fly to China. Poor planning meant his Australian passport was still at the Chinese embassy in Sydney awaiting the issue of a visa. He wouldn't be able to leave without it. But with unbendable determination, he left Australia for Hong Kong on his Dutch passport. Without the required visa, he was denied entry to China. On top of this, his Dutch passport no longer had a valid reentry visa for Australia. I called the Australian immigration department, which confirmed that without it he would not be able to return home. As I expected, I received an email from Dominic in Hong Kong saying he was stranded. He couldn't get into China and he couldn't board a plane and return home. On the advice of the Australian immigration department, I couriered his passport to an office at the university in Hong Kong—the safest option, as Dominic had not provided me or his university department with any other contact details. I did not know where he was staying, when he might enter China, or when he would return home. I'm not sure he even knew himself. At my insistence, he had a mobile phone with him these days but he wouldn't, or couldn't, use it, so I was unable to speak to him. I relied on email, some of which he answered and some of which he didn't. I heard nothing for days and then on my birthday, I got a message.

Happy birthday beautiful, I love you.

He was gone for two weeks. Relieved when he finally got home, I put to rest the visions of the various headlines that had been rolling around in my imagination: "Australian Academic Missing in China"; "Australian Academic Found Dead in China"—and, as I imagined Dominic an easy target, graciously yet unwittingly helping some drug dealers carry their bags through customs en route home, "Jailed Australian Faces Possible Death Sentence."

I rescheduled the appointment he had missed with the neurologist. He came home in time for the psychiatrist's appointment, but I can't remember how on earth I got him there. And I went to see the powers that be at the university.

I drove to the campus, feeling like a reluctant spy trying to maintain the required detachment while at the same time trying to manage her vulnerability. Dominic continued to think his visit to any doctor was a waste of time. And from a medicolegal point of view, the doctors couldn't enforce assessment as Dominic still "fell too much in the gray." But his employers could act on different grounds.

I really didn't want to go this route. I had hoped Dom would agree to medical treatment and retain some professional dignity, but he was planning another trip to Vietnam, and every overseas trip was more dangerous for him. He was in no state to travel. He was deteriorating and seemingly unwilling or unable to use this crisis as a springboard to recovery. Dominic was clearly suffering from something, but unless he cooperated, I faced the possibility that nothing would change until he hit rock bottom and something awful happened to him before anyone could intervene. I emailed my dad.

I don't know what it will take to get Dominic to accept help. I've been banging my head against a brick wall trying to force him to get better and hoping we can get our old life back. It sort of feels like I am dancing the fandango while balancing forty plates on my head and singing "The sun'll come out tomorrow."

I suppose letting go is a process. It is in my nature not to give up until all avenues are explored. Maybe I just need to go through all the possibilities until I know inside myself that searching for any more answers…isn't the answer.

I sat in the HR office of some university tower, feeling conspicuous in my act of betraying Dominic in the hope that it would save him. I also feared disciplinary action from his department—I didn't know if he was getting himself into trouble at work. How do you ask your partner's boss about that? I wanted him to be protected, and at the same time I worried that I would be misunderstood as a dramatic spouse bringing domestic problems to work. Even in the light of all the clear and obvious facts, there were still times I doubted my own perceptions. Regardless, I knew with certainty that the university would be bound by a duty of care to act on the information I was giving them. I would tell them everything. There was no other choice.

"Intuitively," said the head of HR, "what do you think is going on?"

"I'm not sure."

My fears were not established fact, and I didn't want to jeopardize Dominic at work, especially if he could get better. But he needed to be medically assessed and he had to be stopped from going on his next trip to Vietnam. He was not safe and he was a liability to the university. Alongside the stories I had already shared, it was clear that Dominic was becoming more easily confused. He struggled to follow directions and he got lost all over the place. He was the recipient of a prestigious grant, and I worried about his ability to manage the funds. He had increasing difficulty learning new tasks or following complex threads of thought, all of which put him at more risk in another country.

He knew I was at the university, but he thought I was telling them off for bullying him.

I heard the dim sound of a phone ringing in another office down the corridor. When the HR man put his pen down, we talked some more—wrapping-up kind of talk, next steps, clarifying my contact details, a reassuring smile.

"Thank you for coming in." His voice was kind. "I imagine this must have been very hard to do."

We shook hands and I left the building, imagining the immediate phone calls that were being made from behind the closed door. I walked out into the glare of the Brisbane sun and opened the car door to a whoosh of escaping heat. I'd forgotten to put the sunshade up across the windscreen and the steering wheel was too hot to touch. I turned on the ignition and waited for the air conditioner to provide some relief. At least Dominic would now be thoroughly assessed, and I had done everything I possibly could to keep him safe. But I still waited for the shit to hit the fan. I did not know how this would play itself out, but if things had to hit rock bottom before

Dominic could get help, it would be better for that to happen here in Australia than in some jail in Asia.

The university immediately blocked the issuing of air tickets and travel funds. They insisted a full risk assessment be done and scheduled a meeting with Dominic.

"Ask them to dumb the meeting down," the psychiatrist advised me. "Keep it low-key and nonthreatening. We want to avoid a critical incident."

With this advice, the man from HR and the head of department had a casual chat with Dom about needing full medical clearance for staff travel and asked for his permission to be in contact with his doctors. Dominic agreed. As far as he was concerned, he was in great shape and keen to do whatever was needed to head out to Vietnam. He came home talking about this next trip and about the repeated idea that he might resign. He'd go out on his own or move to Vancouver. I worried that an impulsive resignation could leave him unemployed and without insurance benefits should he be put off work on medical grounds. But as soon as Dominic consented to his doctors' talking with the university directly, the issue was flagged with them and Dominic was deemed medically incapable of making a decision to resign. He was protected.

Dom never spoke of what it was like for him on these overseas trips until a poignant lucid moment much later. By the time he had returned home from his travels, things like missed flights or getting lost had dissolved into nonevents for him. His disintegrating brain left him with no carryover effect and no memory of how frightened he must have felt in the situations in which he found himself. As a result, he had no sense of the risk in traveling again.

In the months that lay ahead, he would be diagnosed, he would be medically retired, and he would continue to talk about his travel plans to Vietnam. The doctors would tell me that as the disease progressed, he would become less impulsive and would lose the initiative to act on his thoughts.

In time, he did calm down and our sweet Dominic returned. His passports were hidden and I never challenged his plans. I learned not to worry and to simply say, "Vietnam is lucky to have you, Dom. What is it that you are most proud of?" He would engage, and talk about the things that were important to him. He would do this with a smile, but with limited language, and he would get his facts confused. This nonconfrontational approach allowed us to see the things that still mattered to him and genuinely join him in his sense of accomplishment.

This would not happen for a while yet. Life was still playing out like a thrashing garden hose, squirting water in unpredictable directions. Until we learned how to redirect and tame it, everyone continued to get soaked.

Dominic came back home from the meeting on campus having given the university permission to talk with his doctors. He joined me outside on the lawn as I brushed the dogs. Maxi lay on her back, totally relaxed, legs spread wide and with no shame as she opened her belly to the sun. Her tail wagged at the sound of Dominic's voice.

Dominic went over to Jessie. He stroked her behind her ears with both hands. She licked his face exuberantly before rolling over for a tummy rub. He sat down on the grass with her and laughed, wiping his face on his sleeve. Dominic's relationship with Jessie was affectionate and uncomplicated. She lay on her back, shaking her leg in pleasure as he rubbed her tummy. I handed him her brush. He was easily distracted. In time, I would develop this art of gentle distraction into a finely honed skill.

I became particularly good at diverting conversations away from the inflammatory topic of money. By now, I had invoked my enduring power of attorney and frozen all of Dominic's credit cards. I took over management of our finances, changed the Internet passwords of our bank accounts, and opened a new account in my name from which Dominic could not access our money. Had it really come to this—locking him out of our finances? Going behind his back to save us? Was I Apate or Soteria? Was this deceit or care?

Dominic had become a perfect candidate for exploitation both on his travels and back at home. His lack of comprehension made him a telemarketer's dream. He enthusiastically said "yes" to holidays, charities, and credit cards, generously splashing out money to anyone who phoned or approached him. Given the extent of his inexplicable spending, we were headed for certain financial ruin. We were no longer able to pay the mortgage or the school fees, let alone our everyday bills—the phone, electricity, petrol, groceries for growing boys—and there was no way we could pay off the massive debt that had accumulated. We were in serious financial trouble, and we stood to lose our home.

Dominic had no sense of this, and by now I had stopped trying to get him to understand. I left a little money in our original joint account so that he could use the debit card independently and feel like he had some control. Dominic never knew his finances were being managed. He wouldn't have known the difference between $10 and $10,000. If the money in this account ran out, rather than hit the roof about his lack of financial responsibility, I completely agreed with his frustration, knowing our money was safe elsewhere. Eventually, when the ATM became too confusing for him to manage, I slipped a little cash into his wallet so he didn't have to confront the "stupid machine." As Dominic got sicker, the unused bank card that remained in his wallet was joined by an ID card with emergency contact details in case he got lost. With the help of my solicitor, I rewrote my will, made provision for a trust, appointed a new executor, changed my enduring power of attorney, and changed the beneficiary status on my life insurance policies. Legally and medically, Dominic no longer had decision-making capacity. Moreover I wanted to make sure that both he and the boys would be well cared for should I suddenly be knocked over by a bus.

In the meantime, there was living to do, children to get to school, homework that needed doing, and dogs that needed walking.

Dominic and I finished brushing the dogs. They got up simultaneously and shook themselves clean.

"Want to walk the dogs with me?"

"Okay."

Maxi jumped up and darted around us in uncontainable excitement as I got their leashes.

Dominic walked beside me without saying a word. On our way home, the sky scattered warm plump raindrops loosely over us. We made it back to the house in time to watch the big downpour from inside.

I remembered a time in Vancouver when the boys were little.

"Does it ever not rain in this place?" Dominic had said as he looked out of the lounge window of our tiny North Shore basement suite. His tall, strong reflection sparkled back at us as he pondered the weather through the splatters of rain that drummed on our living room window. It was one of Vancouver's wet, wintry days and we had been cloaked in darkness since 4:30 p.m. Short winter days were part of life in this rain-saturated city. The boys were three and four when we moved there from South Africa. Dominic missed Durban's sunshine and the warm tropical downpours that disappeared as fast they came. They never stole blue skies away for long. He left the window to pour us each a glass of wine and joined me by the fireplace, our legs up, facing each other on the worn brown leather couch.

Dominic leaned back against the armrest and started massaging my feet. He was doing his PhD in town planning back then and was the home-based parent during his student years. I worked to support us, and he arranged his university schedule around the boys, who had so much fun with their dad that they were oblivious to my sense of displacement at not being missed at all.

"How was your day?" I asked

"I spent the morning keeping a horde of wild child pedestrians safe."

It had been his turn on the roster for after-school traffic duty at the boys' primary school, where they were in kindergarten and grade one.

"Seriously, they have the attention span of a flea!" He shifted in his seat, trying to get comfortable. "Where are all the cushions?"

"The boys have them. Our bed pillows, too."

Michael and Nicolas were busy building a fort in their bedroom. One end of a sheet was tucked under the mattress of the top bunk bed, leaving the rest to drape over the back of two kitchen chairs. They used a stack of books to weigh the sheet down. Their alcove was stormproof and filled with every cushion in the house, sleeping bags, and a torch each for reading in the dark.

"How about you—a long day at the clinic?"

My stories about life as a therapist at the mental health clinic always interested him. We both worked with humanity, but in different ways, and there always seemed to be bits we could borrow from each other.

"I couldn't do it."

"Do what?"

"I could never do your kind of work," he said. "Especially if it meant I had to see people who didn't have a grip on reality. If someone came to me and said they could see green goblins, I'd have to tell them they were talking nonsense."

"No, you wouldn't."

"I would."

"Well, how would that be helpful?"

"The whole thing would drive me nuts!"

I offered him my other foot.

"It's just that green goblins don't exist. That's not reality."

"The question of their existence is not the issue. It's how you respond to someone who says they see a green goblin that is most important."

He continued to massage my foot and looked at me with his boyish grin. "I know, beautiful. I don't know how you do it. I just don't have the patience." He cocked his head slightly to one side. "But if anything like that ever happens to me, I want you to be the one who looks after me."

10

A black bowler hat with ribbed hatband and bound edge sat on the filing cabinet in the psychiatrist's consulting room. It was the last thing I pictured seeing in a doctor's office. I wondered if he was the tap dancing type, a guy with a rolled umbrella under his arm and a crimson carnation in his buttonhole, splashing color into people's lives. Or had this hat toppled out of René Magritte's self portrait, "The Son of Man," where a human face remained hidden behind the obscurity of a large green apple?

After assessment questions and a detailed gathering of history, the bowler-hat doctor diagnosed Dominic with bipolar disorder.

"But what about his difficulty in understanding some of what we say?" I said. The silhouetted doctor sat facing me with his back to the window as I looked into the glare.

"He presents as atypical," he said.

"And getting lost? And not understanding things like numbers or the spreadsheets he set up for our budget?"

"I know at times you must think he's dementing, but this can happen with bipolar."

He leaned forward in his chair, out of his silhouette, as if to offer comfort. "Bipolar is treatable. I *promise* we'll get Dominic back." His smile was kind and reassuring. "Give the medication time to kick in, you'll see."

I'm not a doctor, so when the psychiatrist said Dominic's presentation was atypical I hung my hope on it. I left his air-conditioned office that afternoon with a handful of pamphlets.

The air remained thick into the evening, sticking to us like plastic wrap. Nic and I sat out on the patio after dinner. The breeze teased us but brought no relief. It shuffled the humidity around, brushing up against us like hot breath. Dominic was in bed and Michael was in his room, sitting beneath a ceiling fan, working on an assignment.

"I don't think it's bipolar," said Nicolas, holding the pamphlets the doctor had given me for the boys. "Dad isn't like the stuff written here. It doesn't fit."

The phone rang, interrupting us. It was a school friend of Nic's, asking him for help on an English literature assignment due that week. Still holding a list of symptoms in one hand, he lifted his feet up onto the table and made a seamless change of gear to help his friend apply the reader-centered approach to *Mao's Last Dancer*. After hanging up, he leaned back into the chair and studied the booklet again, trying to diagnose his dad.

"I'm not going to get my hopes up."

"Why?"

"I can't believe it's bipolar and then find out it's not. I can't lose Dad twice."

With Nic's hope suspended, Dominic started taking the prescribed drugs for bipolar disorder in addition to some other medication that would calm him down. The symptoms did not change over the next few weeks, and Dominic's manic determination to hop on a plane to Vietnam remained unbending. The bowler-hat doctor had deemed him medically unfit to fly, and his passports were hidden, but none of these restrictions made any sense to Dominic. Polite but emphatic, he refused the doctor's suggestion that he voluntarily go to hospital so that things could be checked out more thoroughly.

Dominic insisted that he was just fine, thank you, and he had to get to Vietnam.

Our options were running out. During our next appointment, the bowler-hat doctor talked me through what might happen. He would try one more time to encourage Dominic to go to hospital on his own accord. If Dominic refused, he would have no option but to hospitalize him under the Mental Health Act for involuntary assessment and treatment. He had to act to protect Dominic's personal safety and professional reputation.

Dominic refused. He couldn't possibly go to hospital—he had a plane to catch. The paperwork came out and I was asked to sign the committal documents. Despite knowing that I was helping Dominic, I felt like his jailer.

Dominic had to go straight from the doctor's rooms in Spring Hill, a spot in the city that housed many medical specialists, to the psychiatric hospital, not too far from there. We were told we could go in a cab, but that if he ran off he would be picked up by police. Dominic frowned in confusion at the word police. What did the police have to do with anything? I watched fear dance with rage across his face.

"We'll go in a cab," I said. "There's no need for the police."

The receptionist called a cab as we stood at the counter in the waiting room.

"You fucking fascist!"

A painfully thin teenage girl moved closer to her mother, her bulbous eyes looking alarmed as Dominic berated me. The receptionist looked up and, in a lowered voice, suggested we wait outside. No one asked if I would be okay out there alone with him.

I had previously made the decision to travel by bus with Dominic to his appointments with the bowler-hat doctor. He became agitated by this doctor who said he couldn't travel, and there was no telling if he would be volatile in the car, making it unsafe to drive without extra help. Now we stood on the sidewalk near a coffee shop with outdoor tables tucked in under a striped cream and brown awning. Its unpretentious charm contrasted with the row of rather bland medical buildings behind it.

"You fucking Nazi!" he yelled at me above the din of the traffic.

"You are just like John Howard! Fucking fascists, the whole lot of you! I'm still going to Vietnam!"

Astounded coffee drinkers stared up at us from their conversations.

A professional-looking woman in a tailored gray pantsuit brightened up with a pink and purple scarf turned around to look at us. She caught my eye and immediately diverted her look elsewhere. I could hear the click-clack of her high heels slapping the pavement as she walked away.

"Fascist!" Dominic said. "I'm going to Vietnam!"

She walked a little faster.

This was not Dominic. If he had known what this *thing* was making him do, he would have been truly mortified. I watched the Green Goblin take over. I didn't challenge him. That always made things worse.

"Fascist!"

He ranted and raved as he paced frenetically back and forth along one of his short, invisible lines, but he was not being physically aggressive.

A man sitting under the awning shuffled in his chair. "It's okay," I mouthed to him. *Stay calm*, I willed the stranger. He lowered himself back into his chair and kept his eyes on us. I kept my distance from Dominic so he had the space to protest and stride safely until the taxi arrived.

"Dom?" I said as it pulled up at the curb. I smiled, offering him my outstretched hand. I hoped I was detached enough from my own pounding anxiety that he could not feel it. Shoulders forward, he came and placed his hand in mine like a dependent child. I helped him into the car.

"Hello!" he said to the driver with a broad smile as he fastened his seatbelt. "How are you?"

"Good, thank you, sir. I didn't know if I had to come up and help anyone. I was told it was urgent."

"Nah, it's not urgent."

Dominic chatted as the driver pulled away from the curb and did a quick U-turn. He sat calmly in the backseat with me, and I noticed how little muscles flickered under his skin, on his arms and across his calf.

I looked out the window, beyond the gawking onlookers and toward the Old Windmill a little further up the hill. Built by convicts, it is said to be the oldest surviving building in Queensland.

Fifteen minutes later, we arrived at the hospital, contemporary prisoners in a world far removed from sidewalk cafés. We paid and thanked the cab driver. Dominic wished him a good day before he drove off. *Please come in with me.* I was having more and more of these internal conversations. Dominic took my outstretched hand as we stepped onto the conveyer belt of medical investigation. There we were, standing still yet moving forward into a sterile world of medical language, tests, and anxious uncertainty.

In his book *The Wounded Storyteller*, Arthur Frank quotes Susan Sontag saying, "We are each citizens of two kingdoms: the kingdom of the well, and that of the sick. Although we all prefer to use only the good passport, sooner or later, each of us is obliged, at least for a spell, to identify ourselves as citizens of that other place."

We had well and truly arrived there.

A young doctor approached us as we entered. Her long, shiny blue-black hair swung loosely over her shoulders with a deep kink. It must have been tied up earlier in the day. She walked through the waiting area of comfy chairs, coffee tables, and magazines to greet us. The light of the sky filtered through the many glass windows and an outdoor courtyard, landscaped with tropical plants and private seating areas, beckoned us from the main entrance. Some thought had gone into reducing psychological barriers to entry here.

"Hi, my name is Dr. Chen. I'm the registrar here today." She had a calm voice and invited Dominic away from the bustle of the reception area, leaving me to fill out all the forms. As they walked down the corridor making small talk, Dominic's gait seemed a little stiff. Signature after signature was added to his chart, and then I waited. I sat on one of the comfy chairs with no interest in reading a magazine. The doctor would see me soon, I was told. They would like a full history of events from me.

I'm not sure how long I sat there before I heard a familiar voice greet me by name. It was the neuropsychologist who had seen Dominic at home a few months before. I wasn't expecting to bump into him here.

He was just as surprised to learn of Dominic's admission. The waiting room was empty. He sat down and listened to the update of events.

"He doesn't belong here," he said, stroking his knee with one hand.

He was certain Dominic did not have bipolar disorder or any other psychiatric condition.

"He needs to see a neurologist, and I'd like to do more tests."

He said he would discuss his concerns with the assessing doctor.

"I'll arrange a referral. I think we are looking at something organic."

I bargained with him about the symptoms. Surely bipolar was a possibility? I knew it was a wretched illness, but it was treatable, wasn't it? If this was organic—and since we already knew there was no brain tumor—the D word was looking more and more likely. I tried everything I could to fend off that diagnosis. Dominic was just too young.

The neuropsychologist sat with me for a while in the waiting room before leaving to follow things up. Time tumbled relentlessly forward, and the day ahead saw me meeting with several doctors, bringing in clothes and some home comforts for Dominic, spending time with him in the leafy courtyard between numerous assessments, and collecting the boys from school before telling them their dad had been admitted to a psychiatric hospital involuntarily.

Later that same evening, Dr. Liam phoned me at home. I was fine until his call. His kindness dislodged my tears as I relayed the events of the day. He reassured me that I had done the right thing, that Dominic was safe now. He could be fully assessed, and we needed the break. When the call was over I lay on my bed, a tide rising inside me. Grief-filled waves rolled out onto my pillow, splattering sadness, emptying me out.

A few days later, the boys and I went to the hospital at about 5:30 p.m. for our first family visit. We entered the warmly decorated hospital, where nurses smiled cheerfully and wore regular clothes, only to find Dominic in the dining room, slowly shuffling forward, part of a dinner line of people that were making their way toward the serving counter. Stooped over and clutching his empty plate with both hands, he was patiently waiting his turn to be served. He looked up at us with vacant eyes and nodded blankly. He was removed from our world and slipping ever further away. I saw Nic watching Dominic and heard the groan of distress expelled from his core. This scene played itself out to me in slow motion, accentuating every detail of the assault on Nic's spirit. No amount of clever interior design was going to disguise what he saw, or soothe the impact of this image on him. The dad he remembered had been stripped of his individuality and reduced to shuffling obediently in line for his food.

I think we all took that image to bed with us that night but none more so than Nic. He still considers this one of his "saddest days ever."

I sat on his bed and watched his sleeping face. Wrapped in the dark folds of the night, he lay in his dreams. A child loved and hurt by a dad locked up and disappearing. I kept him out of school the next day. We hung out or we didn't, we talked or we didn't, and sometime during the day, when the time felt right, we went back to see Dominic.

Michael filled up the dogs' water bowls before we left, and I collected a few things to take to Dominic. I was first to the car and dropped the latest *Manchester United* magazine onto the backseat along with my bag. The driver's seat had been shifted back. Michael, who was growing taller by the minute but remained stripped of weight, must have driven the car last. I fiddled with the lever under the seat and moved it forward. I adjusted the rearview mirror, having a quick peek at myself first.

I looked older than I remembered, and those dark circles, now familiar windowsills to my eyes, could no longer be hidden, even under makeup. The boys were still in the house doing their usual dawdle. I turned on the ignition and was blasted by the screams of some tortured metal band.

I switched it off in search of quiet. Maxi came running out the side gate, wagging her tail and wanting to come along for the ride. Nic took her to the back garden and secured the gate. The boys locked the front door, hopped into the car, and immediately put the music back on.

Life can bring many surprises, but I never thought we would be visiting Dom in a psych hospital.

"We'll put him in the room closest to the nurses' station so we can keep an eye on him—you know, in case he tries to abscond," the admitting nurse had said to me over the top of her reading glasses on the day of his admission. The music in the car drowned out any possibility of conversation with the boys so her words replayed themselves to me through the sounds of our dual life.

"We put the more difficult cases there."

So, he's a "case" now? When did that happen? Just when exactly do you change from being a person to becoming a "case"?

Mike turned the music down as we drove into the hospital's small parking lot. The empty bays were reserved for doctors. There were no bays left for visitors. Obediently, I drove out to find a place alongside the other visitors who had parked out on the street. Not long ago the jacarandas here would have thrown a wash of purple across the road. The shady spots under the now bloomless trees were all taken. I parked in the sun and fitted the sun protector across the front windscreen. Nic picked up the magazine and together the three of us walked back through the parking lot and into the hospital.

I had timed this visit away from any hospital meals or dining room lineups. We found Dominic in his room and made our way to a private spot outside in the garden courtyard. A young woman walked by wearing blue jeans and an oversized T-shirt. Her sunken green eyes sat in a face that had lost its ability to smile. She stared at us intently before walking on. Nic stood very close to me. When she was gone, he gave Dominic the magazine and Mike handed over some of Dominic's favorite music along with earphones. Dominic put them on and smiled as the music we could not hear played. He kept them on, disregarding our conversations as he nodded in time to the music.

Nic paged through the magazine with Dominic. He reached up, took an earphone out of his dad's ear, and said, "You okay? What's it like here?"

"Everyone here is nuts," Dominic said.

Nic put the earphone back in place and watched Dominic's smile reemerge with the music. They continued paging through the magazine showcasing their favorite team. We ate junk food, talked about what sport the boys were playing over the weekend, and made no demands that Dominic engage. Before we knew it, the boys and I were laughing at some rank joke that had been passed along at school. When it was time to go, we put a family photo of us smiling through palm trees at the beach beside Dominic's bed. The boys hugged and kissed him. I asked them to wait for me outside at the car. Mike looked at me with a smile of understanding that could have been Dominic's. He knew how this goodbye might unravel.

"Come," he said to his younger brother. "Let's go, bro."

Once the boys were gone, I picked up my bag and got ready to leave.

I put my arms around Dominic, holding him as, wide-eyed and powerless, he pleaded with me.

"Marie, please, just get me out of here. Please!"

His wrenching words reverberated through my head for days.

He watched me through a window as I walked outside to the boys.

The boys' head of house at school said a lovely thing to me the other day, I wrote to my dad, sister, and brother, when the boys were in bed. *"When it feels like you have lost Dominic, just look at your boys. He is reflected back to you in them. You have two amazing young sons and both of you have contributed to that."*

I lost track of time as my writing transported me to a quieter place.

I can't remember where I read it, but I like the idea that, as my children, Mike and Nic embody all in life I hold dear and true. They reflect pieces of all those I have ever loved. Dom is part of that. I am letting go of trying to control any outcomes and I suspect the news will not be good. Life seems full of hellos and goodbyes right now—so much holding on and letting go.

Dominic had been in hospital for a week and the boys were away. Nic was in New South Wales playing in a school basketball tournament, and Mike was up the coast for a few days with our neighbors, Felicity and Christian, who live over the back fence. Our two families enjoy a kibbutz-type friendship, happily sharing pantries, lawn mowers, spare rooms, and pseudo-adoption of each other's children still living at home: my two boys; Jack, Mike's closest friend at school; and Disa, the sister the boys never had. Felicity and I have nominated each other as crying buddies in sad times, and Christian makes the most scrumptious roast lamb, good enough to tempt even the most steadfast of vegetarians.

It was a Friday night. I came home from the hospital to a house that felt unusually quiet. I didn't feel like dinner and it was nice not to have to cook. A surge of despair whooshed through the silence looking for me, searching for a way to suck me into a vortex that, like a spinning color wheel, spun so fast it would have all the colors of the rainbow disappear into nothingness.

I walked through to the garage, where despair was less likely to engulf me. I opened my box of paints and searched through the half-squished tubes that had once splashed color onto the many canvases now stashed up against the wall. When we had first moved into the house, Dominic had cleared a spot in the garage for me to paint and draw. Never did I have a more avid supporter. When we moved to Brisbane, he had been fully behind the plan for me to work part-time so that I could go to art school. It would be great, he had said. I'd supported him when he did his PhD in Vancouver, and now it was my turn. I could build up a portfolio and start writing and illustrating all those children's books I talked about. Dom loved every piece I did, even the crap ones.

I picked up a cadmium red with an imprint of my thumb pressed into the tube from the last time I had used it. I opened the lid. Red paint oozed out like blood.

I reached for a blank canvas. Trails of red paint followed my fingers as I stroked my hands over it, wondering what my imagination might conceive here. I lugged the canvas and easel, along with the rest of my paints, through to the family room where the light was better. I poured myself a glass of wine, prepared a palette of color, and started filling the canvas with nothing in particular—splashes of color and brush strokes, bold and dripping, to the evocative rhythms of Vangelis.

I turned the music up and remembered the fun I had had with an old art teacher back in my uni days when I was doing art on the side. She was a dynamo of a woman with a mop of red hair that matched the flame of her spirit. She was known for her ability to inspire confidence in even the most insecure of students, so the classes in her home-based studio were always full. *The nude, remember the nude!* Before I knew it, I had shed my clothes and was following the homework instructions she had given us after one of her classes back then.

Paint background on canvas or paper. Strip down naked. Generously smear body with Vaseline. Press body onto prepared canvas to make Vaseline print. Clean up. Get dressed. Pour liquid acrylic paint over canvas. Throw, splash, spray, be wild and spontaneous. Be free, make a mess. Paint will not fix over Vaseline. Once paint is dry, dissolve Vaseline with turpentine. Rub canvas back. Tada! Wonderfully imprecise print of a body will emerge. Rework and build up with charcoal, paint, or whatever you feel like.

Except this night I skipped the get-dressed-again part. There was no need. I was home alone. There I stood, under the downlights in the family room, my naked body sparkling with blue paint and Vaseline.

I propped the canvas on the easel. Holding a glass of red in one hand and wielding a paintbrush in the other, I moved with the music, working up magical markings and accentuating the delicious distortions that were born from my body print. I stepped back to ponder the developing piece. I tilted my head sideways and, as I shifted my weight to one leg, noticed my naked reflection still moving to the music, dancing back at me from the glass panes of the sliding doors that led out onto our outdoor patio and garden.

Then, horror…

The blinds! I had forgotten to close the blinds!

There I was, providing first-class entertainment to our other neighbors, who had guests over for a meal on their patio. Elevated on the upper side of our sloping street, they had a perfect view from their house. The lilly pillies planted at the edge of our garden had not yet grown tall enough to provide a leafy green screen for privacy, and my stunned audience could be forgiven for wondering if the wrong person in this family had been admitted for a psych assessment. I didn't wait to see who was gaping or laughing—paintbrushes went flying along with tubes of paint and the jar of Vaseline as I scampered to hide my glistening body behind the kitchen counter, out of sight.

It was the source of gut-busting hilarity when I relayed the story to a colleague at work the following Monday. We were driving back to the community health center after a home visit to a client when my ringing phone interrupted our spontaneous guffaws.

"Hi, it's Dr. Chen," said the registrar from the hospital. Her voice was upbeat and practical, as though she was passing on a message to a colleague. "Just wanted you to know we've had some results and Dominic doesn't have bipolar. It's nothing psychiatric. It's organic... scans...significant degeneration...frontal lobes...don't know the cause...more tests...dementia...muscle fasciculations...early amyotrophic process...." The words turned to "blah, blah, blah."

I remember not remembering anything.

I remember clearing my head and knowing there was a better way to give bad news.

I remember leaving work and driving straight to the hospital, asking to speak to the doctor directly.

"Hi, Marie," she said, wiping crumbs from her mouth. I had interrupted her lunch.

"Hi, Dr. Chen."

She called me Marie—why didn't I call her Lea? Had I accepted the lower rank of patient's wife?

"Come in," she said. I followed her back into an empty room. "Take a seat," she said as she closed the door. Her voice was kinder and more considered than her earlier phone voice.

I sat down on a steel chair adjacent to the desk and heard the air expel from the plastic seat padding. She swiveled her chair to face me, our knees pointing toward each other. Her black pants led down to a pair of flat red patent leather shoes. The shiny linoleum floor was spotless, anchoring the reflection of her legs into its depths.

I curled my right leg up under me and sat on it as if to spare myself the same cemented fate. The walls that reached up from the floor were bare except for a loudly ticking clock that ran ten minutes fast. The sheets on the examination table were wrinkle free, a contrast to the clutter of paperwork on the desk. A ballpoint pen lay askew, waiting to document the details of the next case.

I liked her, and I did not want to end up in a case note labeled "difficult wife of patient." I would have much less ability to advocate for my family then. Was giving me the news over the phone an oversight of an overworked registrar? Thank goodness I had not been driving. Was she nervous? Or did she chat in clinical speak like she would to a colleague because I was articulate and worked in the health field? I wasn't a health professional in this story. I was a wife with two kids who had just been told on the phone that her husband was dying.

"I'm sorry to just turn up here," I said, "but...can you please go over this with me again?"

"I wondered if you would come by," she said, nodding.

"It's just that I was at work and in the car with a colleague when you called. It was hard hearing it that way."

"I know....I realized when I put down the phone that I didn't ask if you could talk..."

"I know there is no easy way to give bad news. It must be one of the tougher parts of your job, but right now I might need to ask you the same questions a hundred times over. Please let me do this as many times as I need to until I have wrapped my head around what you have just told me."

She nodded again.

My heart became the loudest thing in the room. It thundered over my hope and rattled through my questions. Every now and again I could hear that stupid clock on the wall as, finally, I was introduced to the Green Goblin by name. Dominic had a progressive neurodegenerative illness. The neurologist had diagnosed fronto-temporal lobar degeneration, a type of dementia, with an early amyotrophic process.

There was no cure.

"Does he know?"

"Yes, I spent some time with him this morning."

"Does he understand?" I wished they had waited for me to be with him.

"I think so, although at times it's hard to know."

It was generally difficult to work out what Dominic understood and what he didn't. Lack of insight is an unforgiving trait of this particular type of dementia. It had developed early on for him. In the earlier days, when we had no idea he had a brain disease, we had struggled to understand why he was being so difficult and inappropriate. Now, here in the hospital, talking with the doctor against the sound of a ticking clock, I learned that Dominic was incapable of fully acknowledging the reality of his impairments, that this anosognosia was a symptom of his illness.

In the days to come, I would talk to more specialists and read everything I could about this Green Goblin. Dominic might not anguish like we would over what he was losing, but the very real difficulty was that his lack of insight would make any attempts to adapt to or handle the situation so much harder for him. The frontal lobes are crucial to a person's functioning. They perform all the executive tasks of the brain.

In his book *The Executive Brain: Frontal Lobes and the Civilized Mind*, Dr. Elkhonon Goldberg says these lobes are to the brain what a conductor is to an orchestra. Without a conductor, my Dominic's orchestra was very out of tune.

I sat with Dr. Chen, digesting the news.

"Does Dominic know you are here?"

"Not yet, I wanted to see you first."

"I'm sorry to be giving you such bad news."

I nodded through my sorrow.

"I'll let the consultant know I've spoken with you."

"Thank you," I said, my voice turning to dust by the changing shape of hope. I took a deep breath and went to find Dominic.

The corridors seemed much longer that day. Dominic was in his room. It had two beds. He shared a room with a stranger. He introduced me to him as his beautiful wife. The man remained silent.

"He never talks to me," said Dom as we left the room. "He tried to kill himself."

The haunted green-eyed girl walked past. Dominic turned and followed her like an adoring puppy dog that, even when shooed away, wags its tail and bounds back affectionately for more. I went after him.

"Come, Dom, let's find a shady spot," I said, and took his hand. "You can't do that," I said when we were out of earshot. "It'll freak her out."

He looked at me, confused, and followed me into the courtyard.

Dominic no longer understood the parameters of social space. He was calmer now and generally friendly but he lacked awareness of the impact he had on others. He stood physically close to people, and his chatter could be overly familiar and disinhibited, even with people he didn't know. No longer protected by the boundaries of inhibition, he was increasingly at risk of being misunderstood.

I sat with Dominic on the courtyard steps. I moved closer and held his hand, stroking his fingers with my other hand. I told him the doctor had talked to me.

"It's all bullshit," he said.

I continued to stroke him. He relaxed his hand in mine, some part of him coming back. I told him I'd be there with him all the way through this, and whatever the bullshit brought, he wouldn't have to face it alone. He looked at me and nodded.

A few days later, after two weeks in hospital, Dominic was discharged. Here we were after three years of chaos, or was it closer to four? This slow descent into a runaway world, so subtle at first, was as frightening as hell.

He would never work again. The consultant said it was better to tell him he was on leave for three months. He did not have the cognitive capacity to understand his medical retirement, and it would cause him too much distress. In three months' time the disease would have progressed, and the issue could be addressed in a way that would best meet his needs then. No one knew he would be dead in ten months.

We had a brief session with his doctor before we left the hospital.

"I'm sorry I gave you such a hard time," said Dominic.

"That's okay," said the doctor. "Just go home and potter, get into your garden or something."

It was a funny thing to say to a young man who was going to die, especially when he had led such a full life and didn't like gardening.

We went home, and paid no attention to the garden. A few weeks later, Dominic and I met with a dementia specialist. At just forty-four years of age, Dominic was now under the care of a specialist geriatrician. I read the neurologist's report again. I had forgotten to ask what an "early amyotrophic process" was when Dominic was in hospital. It was one of the several things that had tangled themselves into unquestioned knots in my bombarded brain that day. The geriatrician explained that, alongside frontotemporal degeneration, Dominic had amyotrophic lateral sclerosis, which is also known as Lou Gehrig's disease or motor neuron disease. I wasn't expecting that news. They were linked: FTD ALS it was called, and ALS would most likely be the illness he would die from.

Our lives slipped further into the abyss of hospital corridors and medical appointments. Dominic had a terminal illness with a wide range of behavioral, linguistic, cognitive, emotional, neurological, psychiatric, and physical symptoms. The disease was a thief and wouldn't spare much. There was no cure. No one person experiences all of the possible symptoms, and there is no set order in which they occur.

The bowler-hat doctor talked about this with me, too. He had moved into new rooms while Dominic was in hospital. I liked how he had arranged the chairs in his office. His desk was against the wall and the chairs adjacent to one another. The desk barrier had been removed. The bowler hat was gone—I missed it.

"I'm so sorry I got it wrong," he said.

"It's not your fault."

"I've learned a lot from you and Dominic."

He asked how the boys and I were doing. He sat in his chair without holding a pen or writing anything down. His kindness reached my tears, and a jumble of thoughts tumbled out with them as I contemplated this new journey we were about to travel. Dominic would not get better. Death was a certain destination, and our Dominic would probably be gone before he even got there.

By now I had researched the Green Goblin, and I knew this particular kind of dementia was hard to diagnose. The behavioral disturbances present before any obvious cognitive or physical decline. It is often missed. Families can be turned inside out or broken apart before finding out what is wrong. The fall down the rabbit hole takes a while and, as the family descends, the afflicted person is often misdiagnosed with bipolar disorder, schizophrenia, or depression.

The bowler-hat doctor continued to meet with Dom and me until these appointments became too difficult for Dominic to manage. While the geriatrician helped with symptom management, the bowler-hat doctor focused on ways to help keep Dominic engaged, particularly with the boys. Although Dom never forgave him for admitting him to hospital, he responded well to these "get-togethers." They would Google the UK football wins and losses, as well as the Springbok rugby games. Medical assessments remained noninvasive and subtle as he monitored Dom's decline and helped me with the transition from partner to carer.

"It feels so controlling," I said one day.

"He needs you to manage his world. You are removing the obstacles that are guaranteed to trip him up."

People with dementia are more vulnerable to the impact of their environment on their well-being. I knew this intellectually, but I was uncomfortable taking charge. Our old ways of relating had changed.

I had stepped up in ways that felt counterintuitive.

"If you were able to talk to Dominic now and ask him what you should do, what do you think he would say to you?"

"I know…"

"You are keeping him safe, Marie. He is so lucky to have you."

It didn't feel that way. This new way of being together was foreign to me. We had always consulted with one another. We had listened, we had laughed, and we had argued passionately as we made big decisions. But here I was, his full and legal guardian. I had to make life decisions for him. I had to become his frontal lobe.

At least we had some explanation. I could see now how, before the diagnosis and before the more obvious cognitive changes, our demands that Dominic sort himself out had added to the problem. I often wonder what it must have been like for him to not understand why we were so upset with him, especially in the early days. With zero insight into his condition and limited capacity to understand his world, our insistence that he behave like the Dominic we had always known created expectations he simply could not meet.

Would I have wanted to know the diagnosis earlier? I don't know. Would it have taken away my "if onlys"? I don't know that, either. What I do know is that the more Dominic disappeared from us, the more visible the problem became—the fuller the emptiness, the clearer the view. When the storm ceased, the haze lifted to a forecast of clearer days with slow and constant drizzle. Alongside all forms of emotional weather, we learned to manage Dominic's environment rather than his behavior so that we could give him the best possible sense of personal success in his vanishing world. In doing this, we carved out a new landscape. We reclaimed him from the Green Goblin and simultaneously released him. And, in this new way of being, we got to see so many of the things about him that did not disappear.

He held on to his strong social conscience. He still stood up for the underdog. He continued to oppose the war in Iraq and he didn't hold back in announcing his political views. He had many friends who envied the freedom of his new, disinhibited language, knowing that they would never be able to get away with such passionate diatribes. Perhaps he spoke for them.

Dominic still loved listening to music.

His smile came back.

He boasted about his sons.

He made us cups of tea.

He showed friends all my artwork and encouraged me to keep painting.

And he still loved his sport. When the Wallabies played the All Blacks, he still supported the Wallabies. When they played the Springboks, his loyalty remained divided, but when it came to the English, he remained emphatic—anyone was allowed to beat them.

11

The bookshelves in my childhood home were stacked with life. Whole walls were covered with books. Books filled with exotic lands, fairies, and flowers with unpronounceable names, and stories of wizards, pirates, and celestial cities. I remember, as a little girl, my dad stroking his fingers along the titled spines of philosophy, travel, and history books toward the storybooks I loved, and pulling out the one I had chosen for us to read together. I had a growing list of favorites—*Charlotte's Web*, *The Land of Far Beyond*, Cicely Barker's poems in *Fairies of the Flowers and Trees*, and *The Wind in the Willows*. Black-and-white portrait photographs of all my grandparents sat on various shelves and a photo of my dad as a little boy sitting next to his younger brother perched in a tarnished silver frame on a horizontal pile of gardening books that were too big to fit upright on the shelves. The faces looked out across the room from their nonmatching frames to a colorful photo wall filled with more candid family snapshots, including one of my dad pulling a coin out from behind Reagen's ear. He played magician at our birthday parties year after year, performing all sorts of "un-find-outable" tricks until my group of girlfriends finally gave up on magic and became more intrigued by boys.

There were some closed-in shelves beneath all the books that housed Dad's prized music system. Each evening, after kissing us three kids goodnight, Dad played classical music. He played Mozart's *Piano Concerto No. 21* a lot. The dreamy melody wafted through to my bedroom as I lay in bed listening to the music echo in his heart, knowing he was missing my mother, who had died when I was twelve. It was a precious private time with her each night before he went to bed.

Alongside being a magician and, in my childhood opinion, *the strictest dad in my school, no, South Africa, no, the whole wide world,* he was a born storyteller. My brother, sister, and I starred as key protagonists in invented lands inhabited by animals that could talk and mystical creatures that kept changing shape. He delivered these tales with witty seriousness, filling them with adventure and peril, but, when his nose twitched, we saw plainly how much he enjoyed his storytelling.

As a child and then a teen, I did not realize the influence of the stories I was absorbing from my dad, nor how this ritual we shared was shaping me. I was a curious child and stepped enthusiastically into the worlds he opened up. Alongside the fantasy and fables were true stories—adventurous accounts of an ancestor from the 1750s who had been a spy, as well as a sad story about the time he and two friends went canoeing down the Zambezi River in Mozambique and one of his friends was killed by a crocodile. I would have been two years old when this event happened. We chatted about what it was like to be a child evacuated from London with his little brother during World War II, not knowing when they would see their parents again; how, at the same time, my mum spent seven years as a little girl in an internment camp in what was then Rhodesia because of her German origins; how he had left England at the age of nineteen and traveled to what would become Zimbabwe; and how, given the losses his English mother had experienced as a result of World War II, she had struggled when she learned her son had fallen in love with a German girl.

As a young child, I would sit wrapped in my dad's arm on the couch in the living room or lie on the colorful Persian rug at his feet and listen to his stories. What Dad says he remembers most are my expressive eyes, unblinking and wide open to all the possibilities this time together would bring. Lying on that rug, I was transported on numerous magical carpet rides.

Many years later, as a grandfather, he passed this same wonder on to Mike and Nic, feeding their eager, little-boy imaginations with stories in which they starred, frustrating them with magic tricks they could not expose no matter how hard they tried, and setting intricate traps to outwit Santa on Christmas Eve. The only problem with these traps was that, working together, they managed to make them foolproof. Being the smallest of the adults, I was then left to perform the kind of feats cat burglars take on when navigating a matrix of infrared beams at high-security art galleries. Every Christmas Eve, I would perform a Catherine Zeta-Jones *Entrapment* stunt through an elaborate maze of booby traps connected by string, which acted as a trip switch if I so much as breathed—all this to deliver Santa's gifts, while Dominic and Dad watched to see if I would be caught.

We remember these times like they were yesterday, and telling stories about them is one of those uniting practices we humans seem to do. Together we laugh, we imagine, and we have fun. We find hope, we pass on wisdom, and we cry. We listen, we find each other again, and we remember. Even now, as I write this down, I feel my dad and hear the sound of his voice.

I have the Persian rug of my childhood in my own living room now and, sitting on it these many years later, I had to tell the boys that Dominic was dying.

Nic sat on a chair next to the oak console that displayed a wedding photo of Dominic and me alongside two hand-carved wooden bowls my dad had brought me from India. He pushed his back against the wall, as if by doing so he might prevent it from crashing down on him. I reached out to him, inviting him over to me. He shook his head in a silent no.

"You know how you and Dad are soul mates?" said Michael from the couch.

I nodded.

"He'll wait for you, Mum."

Oh no, Michael's looking after me.

I opened my arms again, and they simultaneously moved onto the carpet next to me, one on either side, burying their heads in my embrace. I sat propped up against an old leather armchair with the boys in my arms and my chest wet with the tears of our intermingled sorrow.

The three of us sat together on this unforgettable carpet ride, knowing there would be no magical ending. Dominic hung between two worlds. There was no cure. He would get sicker. And then he would die.

They asked frank questions. I answered. They let their pauses fill the silence before asking more questions.

"What happens if I can't remember what Dad was like before?" Nic said. "I don't know if I can even remember him when he was well."

Holding them both, I could feel the weight of their accumulated grief. The actively engaged father of their memories was physically alive but no longer present.

"Do you remember when you were about nine, and Dad and I told you we were going to move from Vancouver to Australia?"

Nic nodded.

"You were so upset you almost threw up. Dad got down on his knees so he was the same height as you, then he scooped you onto his lap and held you in his arms, resting his cheek on your head, a bit like I am doing now..."

"Yeah, I remember that." Nic lifted his head and looked at me with an expression of reconnection, the sort of look that is evoked by an awakening memory. He remembered his dad's hold. There was something tactile about it. I knew then that gathering stories would be important and, right there, on the same rug where I had once sat with my dad as a young girl, the three of us made our first step in reclaiming Dominic.

"Remember in Vancouver, when Dad played soccer with us in the freezing cold?"

"Yeah, at the Gleneagles field."

"And when he joined the karate club so he could learn karate with you?"

"Remember how he taught us to skip pebbles?"

"He was awesome."

"He never managed to teach you, Mom—you *still* throw like a girl!"

"Remember when he barbecued on the deck even when it snowed?"

"Mad dude."

"I liked playing chess with him."

"It was cool when he took us to Ambleside Park so we could watch those old men who always played there."

"They sounded like they were Russian or something."

"I played against one of them."

"That guy let you win!"

"Remember the time Dad was in the parents' relay at sports day—the one with the obstacle race where he had to get dressed up in women's clothes and high heels?"

"So embarrassing—seriously."

"But everyone thought he was cool. They were screaming for him!"

"Still, it was random."

"I reckon."

"Only moms did that race."

"Heaps of dads wanted to do it the next year though."

"Still…"

"Your dad—a trendsetting cross-dresser! Who'd have thought it?"

"I'm glad he stayed home with us when he did his PhD and we didn't go to after-school care. Seems kinda important now."

"He was glad, too. He often said so. You guys kept him young. You know, Dad gave Reagen tips on how to win farting competitions when she was a kid!"

"What!?"

"When?"

"She was eight or nine years old. He even wrote her a note about it. I'll ask her to send you a copy."

"Remember how he wrestled with us?"

"And dangled you upside down by your ankles, proclaiming to the world that you would never defeat him?"

"We have an awesome photo of that."

"Remember when he coached our baseball team?"

"Baseball was *so* boring."

"And when he was manager of the soccer team?"

"He hated collecting the money!"

"Everyone on the team called him 'Big D.'"

"Yeah, 'cause he chucked them all in the pool on our Fiji soccer trip. They tried to push him in. Remember? He was too strong, they couldn't!"

"He was kind of invincible."

"Don't people who get this end up in nursing homes?"

"Yes, angel, most often they do."

That night, as my fingers tapped on the computer keyboard, I told my family about how, after the boys and I had talked, we baked chocolate chip cookies. That I noticed we had spent quite a bit of time silently pounding the dough. How I wished Dominic could have participated in our conversation, but, unlike the Dominic of before, he couldn't. How I had arranged for our good friends Edward and Elizabeth to take him over to their place for the morning, leaving me to chat with the boys in the uninterrupted safety of our own home. I wrote on.

When Ed and Liz brought Dominic back home, they spent some time with the boys while I was with Dom. Ed told them that as things get worse, there might be times I am very sad or super busy tending to Dominic's needs. He said if they are worried about me at all, if they need me but I can't be there in the same way as before, or if they need to talk about anything at all, he and Liz would be there for them at all times of the day and night. I'm not sure what I'd do without them, you know. Liz cried when they left. She said she was struck by the boys' ghostly white faces and the look of knowing death in their eyes.

I started to ask family and friends to share accounts of how they knew Dominic—especially as a dad to the boys—and the impact he had had on their own lives. They could be funny stories, affectionate ones, naughty ones—any ones. Photos would be great, too. We would make a collection of them and put them together somehow.

Together, we remembered tales of Dominic's stand against Sister Eusebius, the wicked Catholic primary school nun who was prone to dishing out sadistic lashings with a steel ruler that made his knuckles bleed. Then there was the Afrikaans teacher who, with her overexposed cleavage and very short skirts, had a class full of boys learning a lot more than a second language. There were stories of Dominic the rugby player, the uni student, the activist, the colleague, the teacher, and the treasured friend. We listened to stories of Dominic the son and big brother, Dominic the brother-in-law, the son-in-law, the uncle and godfather. There were Dominic and Marie stories, tales of Dominic the dad, and stories highlighting what the boys had brought into their dad's life: They kept him young and playful, he had always said. They taught him patience; they kept him real; they reminded him that simplicity was where he found contentment; and they stole all his sleep. He loved to hear them laugh. He said it was contagious and, if they had their mum's smile, they'd be extra lucky, because a true smile can shine through anything and can reach anyone.

The boys, now young men, have kept up with some of these storytellers. They don't tire of the tales. They are accounts of life you can tell over and over with someone because, no matter how often you revisit them, you always feel good afterward; you feel part of something bigger.

They chortle at the same old yarns and laugh at anecdotes of Dominic's rebellion on first meeting my dad, who was rather protective of his eldest daughter. Neither of them made it easy for the other in our early dating years. The boys remember Patrick's mischievous tales of Dom's and my sexual playfulness, even when we were parents, and the time when Dom's mother had walked in on us. "Aahhh, gross, too much information!" their teenage voices had exclaimed at the time. Not cool to imagine your parents enjoying sex!

They continue to love it when people recognize an expression of Dominic's on their faces or comment on how they lean back against a wall, lifting one leg up backward, just as he did.

These stories became a tonic, an antidote to the despair, and a way to *re-member*. Remembering not just as a way to reminisce, but *re-membering* as a way to reconnect with a sense of membership and belonging to something important. Barbara Myerhoff, a cultural anthropologist, talked about this concept a lot in her writing. Her fieldwork with elderly Jewish members at a senior day center in Venice Beach, California, went on to influence the anthropological study of ritual and life histories. She said *re-membering* can be used to "call attention to the reaggregation of members, the figures who belong to one's life story, one's own prior selves, as well as significant others who are part of the story."

Myerhoff, and those like Michael White (cofounder both of narrative therapy and of the Dulwich Centre in Adelaide) who built on her insights, refer to this special type of *re-membering* as an intentional act of connecting to significant others, which links us not just to a sense of self but to a community of belonging that contributes to a "multivoiced" sense of identity.

Our *re-membering* would not save Dominic, but sitting on that carpet we started reconnecting to a relationship with him that became real and visible again. The carpet we were riding had no magic power—we were losing Dominic even before he died—but it would fly us to the places where we could always find him again.

12

I walked into my first meeting at one of the community dementia organizations and was welcomed by the smiling faces of friendly old people looking out at me from glossy posters on the wall. They heard me take a deep breath and look around. They knew what this was like—walking into a place like this for the first time, hoping to find help to manage and adapt. They had been here too, once, although they had been retired when they got sick. Most had grandchildren. They chatted among themselves and agreed that their adult children would probably be about my age now, maybe even older. *You'll be okay,* they smiled. *Look at us, we were helped by this organization.*

Dominic's geriatrician had referred me here in the hope we could access some support. However, we were a completely new situation for them. They'd never dealt with a young family like ours before. There was no one like me on the wall. Even the "early onset" posters sitting above the bookshelves showed people that were much older than us.

"You must be Marie. Are you here for the carers' group?" A young woman wearing a name badge left the photocopying machine and greeted me. "Feel free to browse through the books any time. We lend them out."

She showed me where to get a cup of tea or coffee and then took me through to a room where a group of twenty or so people was gathered.

A couple of spare chairs stood empty between chatting carers. I slid in and found myself a seat. I had no idea what to expect, but my memory of that encounter is now seared into my consciousness. The room quieted as a counselor introduced herself and greeted the gathering.

"Now that you know who I am," she said, "I'd like everyone to introduce themselves and to tell the group who they are caring for. Right, let's start with you…" She lifted the strands of curly auburn hair that repeatedly fell across her face and nodded at the person to whom she had just pointed.

"Hello. My name is Mary, and I'm caring for my mother, who is ninety-one years old."

"Hi, there, my name is Jean, and my husband is in a nursing home. He is eighty-five."

"I'm Shelley. I'm caring for my father Joseph. He is also eighty-five and about to go into care. My mother is in a nursing home, too, but she doesn't have dementia."

"Hi, I'm Marie, and I'm caring for my husband…"

The room fell silent, followed by a collective gasp.

"Yes, he's only forty-four," said the counselor before the gasp had been fully expelled. "It's a bit of a different situation," she added, without looking at me.

"I thought she was here for a parent!" A woman's whisper echoed across the room, bouncing off people's faces until it landed on my lap, pulsating there as their silent thoughts were absorbed into the hum of the air conditioner.

I felt hot under the glare of everyone's attention.

The counselor pulled the unruly strand of hair off her face again.

"And, what's more, they have two young teenage sons!" she said.

Another group gasp circled the room, this one shaped by pity. An image of the counselor sitting in a 1950s hair salon flashed through my mind—her head stuck under a bonnet dryer, that same piece of loose hair bothering her, throwing out snippets of intrigue to the women sitting around her.

"He's had this for a few years, you know. Can you imagine young boys dealing with this—all the trauma?"

She didn't wait for a reply and spoke through the shaking heads and *tsk-tsks* of others. "But I have a lot of experience in grief work and I've offered to give them counseling," she said. "This situation is very complex—yes—especially with boys, as you know. For them to recover, they will need to get their feelings out. It's absolutely crucial."

So, this is the person the organization has offered up as help for my family. This was my first encounter with her; she must have been primed about us by someone else. I had never met or spoken to her before, let alone given her permission to disclose her assumptions about our family to a room full of shocked strangers. Silenced and set apart, I sat under a spotlight of pathologized difference. What impact would "help" like this have on the boys?

I diverted the attention back to the group and slipped out at the first break, deciding to continue with the support I had already found for the boys and me elsewhere. I walked past the friendly poster people as I left the building. If they were able to read my thoughts, they would know of my hope that the boys could have a different story about themselves at this time in their lives than had been offered up here. One in which they would know themselves as loved, wise, resourceful, courageous, and graced with a great capacity to love.

I headed for the car, thinking through the most helpful way to give this agency my feedback. I had parked around the block. Parking is always difficult in the city, but on this day in particular, I was glad of the chance to walk before battling city traffic.

The drive home was smooth and uneventful. Half an hour and a world away from salon gossip, I walked through our front door.

"Hey, Mom, is your camera charged?" said Nic.

"I think so."

"Can you take some photos?"

"Sure, angel. What for?"

"You'll see." Nic went to the bathroom and got out Dominic's shaving gear and an extra razor.

"Hey, Dad, wanna teach me how to shave?"

Dominic was in the family room. He made his way over to the bathroom.

"It's a novelty shave. I know I don't have any hair yet," Nic whispered to me.

Nic's eyes looked back at me from the bathroom mirror. They reflected a sad knowing, delicately framed in a young boy's face without a wisp of facial hair. His dad would never see him grow into a man. He so wanted to know this moment, and while he claimed for himself this father-son experience, he also gifted Dominic with another opportunity to be his dad.

Memories of my young mother flooded me. She had wanted to buy me my first bra—one last act of motherhood before she died. I was twelve and still as flat as a pancake when breast cancer took her from us. She was in obvious pain, but insisted my dad take us bra shopping. The irony was lost on me then, but while wearing her prosthesis she found me a pretty white bra with a little pink rose in the center: a symbol of hope for the daughter she would not see through puberty.

"Do you remember shaving with Dad as a little kid?" I said as I started to take photos of Nic with Dominic.

"Sort of, not really."

"I do," said Dominic. "You were little…in Vancouver. You and Mike shaved with me every day. I gave you…?" He held out the razor he was using, searching for the word.

"A razor?" said Nic.

"Yes...no..." Dominic looked at me.

I leaned against the doorway, smiling at the memory. "You took out the blade."

Dominic nodded and grinned at Nic.

Every morning, little four- and five-year-old Mike and Nic had stood on tippy-toes with their white, frothed-up chins barely reaching the top of the vanity. Using bladeless razors, they had earnestly joined Dom in his morning shave.

Nic was now a whole lot taller. Two fresh-bladed razors lay on the counter. Dominic wet his face with warm water. Nic did the same. He squirted shaving gel onto Nic's fingers, then his own, and together they applied it across their faces and under their chins using small circular motions.

"Shave the way the hair grows."

Nic nodded.

Dominic shaved downward from his sideburns along his jawline toward his chin. Nic followed, exposing a fresh track of young skin. Dominic ran his razor under a running tap to unclog the blade and moved aside for Nic to do the same thing. As they moved forward, they pulled their skin taut with their free hands and continued the shave. Standing sidebyside, real Gillettes in hand, their arms moved in unison over their cheeks. Soon they were each left with a white moustache. They rinsed their razors again, curled their top lips over their front teeth, and shaved their whiskers into the waiting camera with small, gentle strokes.

Dominic started to sleep with a baseball bat under his bed. He placed it carefully, in just the right spot, an arm's reach away, checking several times that it was still there. The first time he did this, I took the bat away.

"No, I need it!" he said.

"What for?"

"How would I protect you if burglars broke in?"

"Are you worried about burglars?"

"This place is so easy to break into. They would probably come right through that window." He pointed to our bedroom window, which, in all fairness, was probably the first window any burglar would try if they wanted easy entry.

"Promise me you will never sleep with that window open if I'm not here?"

"Okay, I promise. But couldn't you protect me without the bat?"

"You never know what weapons they will have or how many of them there will be."

"We can always get the bat if the burglars come in. That way we won't have to worry about an accident happening."

"No! I need it under the bed."

There was no persuading him. I handed him the bat. He placed it carefully under the bed and turned off the light. I waited until he was asleep before I opened the windows he had closed to let the cool evening air back into the room. I stood beside his sleeping form and noticed a little frown embedded in his forehead. In the quiet, I could almost hear his brain crackle. He lay motionless on his back with his hands clasped over his chest as if he was praying. I stood out of reach and coughed to see if he would stir. He didn't flinch. I bent slowly, keeping my eyes on him, and very quietly removed the bat from under the bed. I tiptoed away and hid it, learning to make it plainly visible the next evening before he went to bed so we did not have to deal with his fear and agitation at not being able to find it. With the bat out of harm's way, I climbed into bed. I repeated this ritual night after night until one day Dominic didn't look for the bat at bedtime anymore, and he never asked for it again. Dominic never used the bat. He never displayed any aggression with it, either. He was unaware of my anxious anticipation of a potential psychotic flare-up; he simply needed it to go to sleep.

Baseball bats and shaving tenderness lived side by side in what soon became our new normality. I am fortunate that through my work and the research of others in the field, I have some understanding of the ways in which our relationship to illness can affect both how we know ourselves and how others view us.

Kaethe Weingarten, an associate clinical professor of psychology at Harvard, writes about this in detail. People's interactions with the world can be impacted by the various stories we hold about illness, and "anything that helps put illness in its place, that allows us to feel that we are who we are despite it, is welcome," she says.

Once we knew that Dominic had a brain disease, it became easier to understand his behavior. It gave us an explanation for the desolation that had been caused. Life would be very different, but we no longer doubted the history our little family shared together. We were able to start separating the illness from Dominic as a person, and I hoped it would give us a better chance of being who we were despite the Green Goblin's incursion.

Two months after Dom was discharged from hospital, we threw Michael an eighteenth birthday party. Time doesn't wait for Green Goblins.

Life happens simultaneously; there is no pause button. I looked at my baby, now a tall young adult. He had been only fourteen or fifteen years old when life took a different turn, and here he was, taller than his dad and dressed to kill. The theme was black and white. Ed was our "bouncer," and between him, Liz, and my friend Beth, who were core to the community of loving hands and hearts that supported us, we had a team of party organizers, birthday celebrators, and Dominic advocates. The evening was filled with laughter, pumping music, games of pool, and young people who took the theme to a glamorous level of sparkle and sophistication. How did Dominic, the all-out boardies and T-shirt guy, and me, the Indian-cotton girl, produce sons who liked to spruce up?

Dominic jumped at the sound of a popping balloon. Beth held out her hand. He took it. Who would have thought, when I met her at work soon after arriving in Australia, that she would have stepped into my life like this? He was restless and showed signs of increasing fatigue from the overstimulation, but he would not be distracted into bed.

"NO! I DON'T WANT TO MISS ANY OF IT!" he said.

His eyes were wide and emphatic, as if he knew he wouldn't be here for another one. He turned and shuffled outside, shoulders forward, arms dangling loosely, staring blankly through uncomprehending eyes. It could have been disconcerting for the boys' friends, but determined his dad would have a respectful audience, Mike set the comfort radar to "relax." That night, advocacy became a shield against sorrow. He smiled at his dad, put his arm around him, and had no expectations that he engage in conversation or behave in a socially acceptable way. He had spoken to some of his friends before they arrived that night. Dominic mirrored the mood set by his son and paced aimlessly through the crowd, feeling very much a part of it. Nic watched from the garden. He smoothed down his shirt and tucked the sadness back in.

A few of the boys' friends approached me during the evening, asking how Mike and Nic were doing.

"Are they okay? They don't really talk about it," said one friend, leaning against the kitchen counter as I prepared the next tray of snacks.

"Yeah, is there anything we can do?"

I had heard horror stories of drunken eighteenths and police being called to break up wild scenes, but this was very different, other than a few discreet garden-bed vomits. This Gen Y bunch was genuinely concerned. The next morning there was a knock on the door. Joining the few that had slept over, a bunch of blurry-eyed teens arrived to help clean up.

Michael pulled out the ingredients for a greasy hangover remedy brunch and laid them out on the kitchen counter.

"Who's up for bacon and eggs?" he asked.

Grunts of approval followed.

"Nic! You're on the barbecue."

"Hey, why me? You do it."

I took Dominic out for a long drive, away from the smell of greasy breakfast sausages and loud music mixed in with teenage testosterone.

A few hours later, I came back to a place that was spotless and silent.

The bins were overflowing, the floors mopped, and Mike and Nic lay sprawled diagonally across their beds, fast asleep.

A few hours later, Mike woke up. He went to the fridge to pour himself a glass of cold milk, but the carton was empty.

"I've got to drop these speakers back at Mitch's. I'll stop off at Coles and get milk on the way."

Dominic followed Mike out to the car and jumped in the passenger seat next to him. He could not be distracted out of the car. He had refused a shave that morning and, despite the earlier drive, he was disoriented and disheveled. Mike looked at me from the driver's seat.

"I'm fine. Dad likes the drive. It'll relax him," he said. "And I don't care what people think, he's still my dad."

Michael carried a special card in his wallet in case he needed to discreetly show it to anyone who was disconcerted by his dad's behavior. He checked that he had it. It peeked up at him from a cardholder slot with the message: *I am a caregiver of someone with memory loss and confusion. Please be patient.*

Patience, lots of it, lined our days as we learned to help Dominic navigate his slowly narrowing world. Alongside our sorrow, we began to understand the Green Goblin and to relax with Dominic when he did strange or annoying things. Dominic's brain was dying, and the empty spaces started to fill with teaching, honesty, shared tears, and laughter.

A few weeks after Michael's party, Dom's brother Daniel flew in from South Africa with his toddler son. My brother Patrick would be the next to fly in, then our friends from Vancouver. Graham would come first. Grace would come later, they thought, after Dominic died, when I would probably need her most.

We had planned a trip to North Stradbroke Island with Daniel. Straddie was a favorite family holiday spot. Despite his phone conversations with Dominic, and my frequent email and phone contact with Daniel, I wondered how hard it must have been for him to imagine the brother he would meet when he got here. He had not seen Dominic in a year. How does one prepare for such a visit? When Daniel first saw Dominic, he was visibly shaken by his decline. I, somewhat desensitized to the degree of Dominic's deterioration, had been nervous Daniel might not notice anything, that he would confirm that I was being dramatic or exaggerating.

Sometimes Dominic's impairments were not clearly visible to others. Somehow, he held it together more when friends and colleagues popped over. Their short morning visits, when Dom was less tired, did not show the extent of his disabilities. With less and less brain capacity available to him, he put every ounce of energy he had into managing these interactions. When people left he was all used up and there was no Dominic left. People didn't see what we saw or what we lived with. Nic said it made it all invisible and so much harder to feel believed. He didn't talk about Dominic's illness outside of our home. How could he, when it felt like the Green Goblin was making a liar out of us?

"I miss him," he said. "Dad's not alive, and he's not dead either."

Dominic had always loved Straddie. We packed the car full of supplies and beach gear and made our way to the island for a family getaway. Perhaps he would relax here; perhaps we would see more of him. Maybe the ocean would reach him, and we would spot the Dominic that came alive as he bodysurfed and played with any kind of beach ball.

But this time the waves crashed wildly over seven-foot sharks; he could see them. He told the lifeguard, who didn't listen. He walked to the beach, then back to the beach house, then back to the beach, only to turn on his heel and walk home again. I walked with him. He was too confused to be left alone, and none of us could find the off switch. The Dominic we knew did not reappear. Being away from home was increasingly difficult for him.

Dominic's pacing was ghostlike. He made no sound as he floated across the beach house floor. His arms hung rigidly by his side, and he used his feet to maneuver his stiffened body, without a hint of a twist to his waist. We grew eyes in the backs of our heads. The boys latched the front door, hoping it would prevent Dominic's roving, but he became agitated and tried to climb over the patio railing, which was not on the ground level. There was no stopping him. We quickly unlatched the door, and I continued to join him on his determined dementia walks. Through the chaos, over the agitation, to and from the beach all day in a continuous search for stillness.

Just like at home, the Straddie night air brought Dominic no sleep, and his baby nephew's cries reverberated in his head like a gong, pushing him further into agitation. He was on drugs strong enough to knock us all out on one shared tablet, but he was up throughout the night.

He could no longer manage away from the familiarity of his own home.

I knew this would be our last family holiday with Dominic.

On our last night on the island we thought we would do something special. Savoring life in the in-between places, we had a pancake evening. Pancake evenings had been legendary events in Dominic's family as he was growing up. He and his two teenage brothers would sit around the family dining room table eating obscene amounts of pancakes in one sitting, competing to out-gorge each other.

"You guys ate epic amounts," said Mike.

Daniel laughed. "It was pretty epic."

It became evident to him that stories of pancake evenings and supreme domination had traveled down the line and that Michael and Nicolas had also taken part in the Williams pancake challenge.

"How many could you eat in one go?"

"A lot! I don't remember exactly, but I never managed to engulf the quantities Dominic did."

"So, like, take a guess—how many do you think?" said Nic.

"Geez, now you're asking—I dunno, maybe fifteen? Hey, Dom, you reckon I could eat fifteen, or seventeen maybe?"

Dominic smiled blankly.

"Maybe I'll add on a few then!"

The boys laughed.

"I haven't managed that many yet—but the battle's not over," said Nic.

"Dad used to make heaps for us," said Mike.

"It was awesome," said Nic.

"I remember your mum doing that, too," I said to Daniel.

"Doing what?" asked Nic.

"Making huge piles of pancakes. She had a special way of keeping them warm so that the pancakes didn't dry out. She would stack them up on a plate sitting over a pot of boiling water on the stove."

"I know!" said Daniel. "She'd try and get a good pile going before we started eating them. I remember one night, I think we were all still at school, she made more than usual and none of us could believe it—Dominic ate twenty-two!"

"Yeah, Dad told us about that," said Mike, putting his arm around Dominic.

"No one makes pancakes like your mum," I said to Daniel. "Can you match her tonight?"

"Pressure's on!" said Nic.

Daniel placed the ingredients on the kitchen counter. He cracked the eggs into a large bowl. Nic added milk, sugar, and flour, and

Michael added various secret ingredients before proceeding to hand-beat the mixture. There was no electric beater in the unit, so the bowl circulated as arms got tired. There could be no shortcuts. The texture had to be perfect.

We ignored the flour-dusted countertop, broken eggshells dribbling egg white on the floor, and sugar slowly spilling from a tear at the bottom of the package. The mixture was now perfect and ready for flipping in a fry pan.

The first few turned out like sticky Frisbees.

"Don't worry," Daniel said, "the first ones are always flops. They make good snacks."

Daniel and the boys looked keenly for bubbles forming in the batter, drying edges, and golden color. Then came the flip, along with the hope that the pancake would land back in the pan. One or two dangled over the side but were squelched back into the pan, looking more like folded omelets than perfect pancakes. They were cooked up a bit more for another snack. Before long, three jesters were flipping pancakes with circus skill and laughter, preparing for the feast that would follow.

Dominic stopped pacing the room to watch. A smile broke through his confusion. He had lost his sense of taste. He had lost his sense of smell. But he knew what this was about, and the reminiscence was delicious.

To this day, no one has been able to beat his record of twenty-two pancakes eaten in one sitting.

He remains the all-time pancake king.

13

I walked past several posters of missing persons in the front lobby of our local police station and made my way up to the counter. A woman followed me in, talking to herself, complaining about the heat.

"Can I help you?" said a soft-spoken sergeant sitting at the front reception desk.

The woman waited behind me, fanning herself with a handful of official looking forms.

"Would it be okay…um…is there somewhere we could talk privately, please?"

The sergeant nodded. He had crystal-blue eyes that were curtained with thick, dark lashes. He invited me into an adjoining room.

He poured me a glass of water and sat on a chair adjacent to mine. He waited, not rushing me to talk. I told our story. My husband was sick. He was a young man with dementia. For some reason he needed to walk. So we walked and walked. But he had started to wander the streets looking for me when I was at work. I had received a few calls from neighbors filling me in on "Dominic sightings." At first they weren't sure what to do. I had to keep an eye on whether his walks were purposeful or lost wanderings; there was a fine line between keeping him safe and taking away his independence. For now, he didn't wander far, repeating the same route, always making it safely home. The Green Goblin was simply becoming acquainted with the neighborhood. But if Dominic got lost or was found wandering the streets confused, distressed, or "acting strangely," there was an explanation. He was not drunk, psychotic, or misbehaving. He was a young family man, with frontotemporal dementia and amyotrophic lateral sclerosis, who was probably trying to make his way to work or to the airport. It was an unusual situation for a man of this age. People wouldn't necessarily understand if they met him.

I handed the sergeant a photo. For as long as I had known him, Dom had hated being in front of a camera. We often ended up with mug shots or pictures of him frowning, with his mouth open in protest. This one was different. Dominic smiled back at the world in a candid shot he never knew had been taken.

"I'm so sorry you are going through this," said the sergeant. "Please be reassured we have people trained in this sort of thing— I'll get the right people informed straight away." He looked back down at the photo in his hands, at a man of a similar age to him.

I hoped these trained people would never be needed, but if they were, I hoped they would approach Dominic in a way that would be most helpful to him and those around him, especially if police intervention was ever witnessed by Michael or Nicolas. Please, I told the sergeant, no facedown takedowns, no restraints. It would only heighten Dominic's anguish and make everything worse. And I told the sergeant about the boys. They'd been through a lot. Dominic was on medication now, but if things got out of hand like they had before, or if we couldn't find him, we might need to call 000. The sergeant nodded and took down all our contact numbers, including the boys' mobile numbers. He said he would flag us as a priority with the central communications office.

While the sergeant took notes, I explained how Dominic responded best to genuine gentleness. If they had to intervene, the trick was to be kind, cheerful, and calm, and Dominic would usually comply. If he did not feel challenged he could be a placid and obliging soul, even when confused. He loved to talk about his sons and was easily distracted with conversations about sport. If they called me, he would probably come home with me without any trouble. I gave him the doctors' details, along with the name and phone number of the hospital where Dominic had been two months ago. If it were ever needed, he could be accompanied back there, where he was known, and not taken to another hospital where, with no history, he would be zapped with sedatives that would have his unyielding, frightened body slowly soften in strangers' hands. He would be locked up in a psych ward and put through the whole assessment drama all over again, only to have the doctors realize he did not belong there in the first place. An inappropriate admission like this would unleash the beast: increase Dominic's distress, exaggerate his symptoms, and result in a traumatic yet easily preventable event.

The sergeant coded us as a priority, gave me his direct number, and invited the boys and me to call him personally at any time with changes or updates. I took another sip of water and thanked him.

"That's what we are here for," he said.

Another danger neutralized.

I left the station and drove to work. I looked at my watch. Our good friend Jo would be with Dominic by now. I relaxed. I had used up all my carer's and annual holiday leave. Friends popped in to see Dom most weekday mornings; they developed a bit of a roster. This way he could still have meaningful social connections he could call his own, and I could go to work knowing someone was with him for a couple of hours. They walked the dogs, went for drives, and made dinners in our kitchen for when I got home, and they discussed a jumble of politics, including how to end the cycle of poverty, as they looked through photographs of Dominic's projects in faraway places.

Genevieve would be visiting tomorrow. She was the first friend I had made in Australia. Her twin daughters, Chloe and Lilly, were barely six weeks old when she had come up to me at school, noticing

I was a new mum, and invited me over for coffee. The twins were now six years old and our fridge was becoming more and more color- ful as little Lilly's pictures were added to the growing collection.

"When is Dominic going to die?" Lilly had asked me one day.

I told her I didn't know when it would be, but that he was getting sicker. From then on, she started drawing pictures for him.

I imagined a new picture appearing the next day, and Dominic making Genevieve a cup of tea—dunking tea bags in the water and watching the color swirl. He would have two neatly lined up mugs, complete with green vanilla tea bags, waiting on the kitchen counter for her from the time he got out of bed in the morning. Dominic didn't know how to wait for 9:30 a.m. He was losing his sense of time—of the past and the future—but there was always the present. What better time was there to make tea for friends?

I arrived at work and parked in the staff parking lot at the com- munity health center. The bowler-hat doctor and the geriatrician had both said Dominic was safe to be at home alone. He was on medication and, although detached, he was calm. Under no circum- stances was he to make his way to work. Keeping him off campus would help protect his professional credibility, but he didn't need full-time supervision yet, and it was okay for the boys to be at home with him after school if I wasn't there. I got busy with my day: seeing clients, writing reports, and attending meetings, not noticing I was getting thinner, losing part of me alongside Dominic.

The phone rang.

"Mum, Dad's gone!" Michael's panicked voice tumbled down the phone. "He caught the bus to uni! I raced to the bus stop to see if I could bring him home, but he was already on the bus!"

He told me Dominic had asked him to drive him to work.

"I showed him there were no cars in the driveway, so I couldn't do it now. I said one of us could take him when you got home from work. He always waits for you to come home from work. He seemed fine—"

"It's okay, darling—"

"He was cool with it, you know—he wasn't agitated or any-thing—and he came back inside and went to lie down, so I went back to my room and worked on my assignment, and when I came out to get a snack, I found a note on the kitchen counter."

"He left a note?"

"Yes, he's on the bus—what if he gets lost?"

"How long ago did he leave?"

"I'm not sure, I didn't hear him go."

"It's okay. I'll follow the bus route and I'll meet him there. I know where to find him."

"I didn't know…"

"It's not your fault, angel. It would have happened if I was at home, too. It'll be okay."

"He said he wanted to find out why his work email wasn't working and something about going to Vietnam."

"You okay, honey?"

Quiet.

"Mike?"

"This sucks."

"I know. It really does."

Dominic would have to catch two buses to uni, which was prob-ably more than he could manage. I had to hand it to him, he was pretty determined. And that meant this might be one of those times when it was difficult to bring him home. Mike stayed at home in case Dominic returned.

I called Antony, Dominic's head of department, and let him know Dominic was on his way. We had prepared for this possibility a few weeks earlier, when I had met with him and someone from HR to sign Dominic's permanent medical retirement documents.

"Total and permanent disablement" was the terminology.

More documents signing his life away.

Despite his obvious decline and doctors' orders not to do so, I had expected Dominic to make his way onto campus eventually, regardless of attempts to distract him. We were going to have to manage this carefully. The Goblin could put on quite a performance if challenged, and his colleagues did not need front-row tickets for the show.

His doctors had stipulated that he attend his medical appointments, not travel, not drive, and not go onto the university campus. However, Dominic did not understand these restrictions, and this left him vulnerable in so many ways. He struggled to adjust. Why was he told he could not work right now? He had a trip to plan. His PhD students wanted him to continue supervising them. He was an external examiner for a thesis; he had to get on to that. Couldn't the department see he was fine?

"I think they want to get rid of me," he had said to me a couple of weeks earlier.

"No way. You're exhausted, and they want you to rest. You've worked yourself to the ground."

"No, I'm on the second floor."

"Yes, you are, and you know how you said the workload is ridiculous?"

"Yup!"

"I reckon they realize it: the doctors have told them you need a break. It's just three months, remember, and they are giving you time off with pay. Check this out…"

I read him emails from colleagues at the university where warm support had been unambiguously expressed. The place wasn't the same without him, they said. They were keen to visit. They missed him. I didn't use the words sick or sick leave. I'd done that before and learned the hard way that it didn't work. He thought he was fine and, had I argued with that, I would have lost him completely.

Antony and I had kept in regular contact throughout Dominic's unraveling. I remember sitting in his office one morning with a box of tissues thoughtfully slipped toward me in case I might need them. I gave him as much information as I knew about how we might best respond to this goblin, at least while it was still feisty enough to cause trouble. The geriatrician, who was also a professor at the same university, advised Antony about the ins and outs of Dominic's illness, too—what to expect and how to manage things. The safety net, interwoven with kindness and understanding, was slowly expanding.

With Dominic on the bus, Antony and I talked on the phone and went over what to do, but the best strategies don't always work. We all knew that.

"I have it all covered," said a friend at work—the same friend who had been with me in the car when I received the bad-news call from the hospital. "I'll reschedule your clients. Nothing here is urgent."

She was all calm and no fluster, the perfect friend at a time like this. She put an arm around me. "Go. I'll tell the others. Just go. And call me if you need anything."

I left work and picked Ed up on the way in case I needed an extra person to help. We followed the bus route, keeping our eyes open for Dominic, until we received a call from Antony saying he had arrived on campus. We headed straight for the gardens outside the department, where the two of them were chatting about their kids and soccer.

"Hi, mate. We've popped in for a coffee," said Ed.

Dominic gladly followed him to the coffee shop. The sun pushed against the shade as Antony and I stood under the trees in the encroaching heat and talked. Dominic was deteriorating more quickly than we had thought. It wasn't looking good.

The coffee shop did not provide enough distraction. Dominic was not going to come home until he could get his computer to work and plan his trip to Vietnam. He wouldn't budge. He made his way up to his office, to the same desk where brilliant ideas had once been developed. Now Antony, Ed, and I watched him struggle as he tried to log on to the computer.

"You don't need to be doing emails when you are on sick leave," said Antony.

"I'm fine."

"Well, it's policy to close remote access down when a person is off for a while—it makes sure people rest and take the break they need."

"But I need the computer."

Dominic continued reentering his password, which had been blocked.

I dreaded the possibility of a scene on campus.

"Is there any chance you could get hold of the IT guys and just ask them to look at it? We can go for a drive while they're working on it," I said to Antony.

"Sure." Antony nodded, acknowledging the change of direction.

Dominic looked up and smiled. "Thanks."

"It was good to see your office," said Ed to Dominic. "And nice to meet you, Antony."

Fear collapsed and made room for fresh air as Dominic left his desk and joined us in a stroll back to the car. We made our way home, Dominic happy that the IT guys would get to the bottom of things and the rest of us knowing no such call would be made. Regardless, Dom would get home safely without having been compromised at work.

The next day Antony called, checking in on us all. "Jeezus, this is a bugger to manage!" he said. "How are you doing?"

I was so relieved by his spontaneous acknowledgment, validating all of us somehow. The boys were right: It sucked. It really sucked. Antony wondered if Dom was up for a visit. Over the next months, he dropped by quite often. I asked him once when he had first started to notice a change in Dominic at work.

It was hard to say, he said. He couldn't understand the change. "At first, I thought I'd offended him. I thought maybe it was me."

In between Antony's friendly visits to our home and Dominic chatting to him over tea about his next trip to Vietnam, Dominic made a few visits to campus. One morning, Antony called me at work to let me know Dom was in the department. How many times was I going to have to leave work and do this uni dash?

Antony had Dominic roaming the department and me, choking on tears of exasperation, on the other end of the phone. What head of department has to deal with this sort of thing in an ordinary day's work?

"It's okay, Marie. We care about you. We can do this. I'll be here for you both."

Despite the many difficulties he must have encountered with this goblin, Antony kept unfalteringly to his word, even after Dominic died.

Dominic remained preoccupied with plans to travel to Vietnam and a simultaneous quest to apply for jobs overseas. The geriatrician said to expect this might go on for a while. I did not want to interfere in his professional life but, after seeing some of the emails he had tried to write from home, I felt I had no choice. I contacted three of Dominic's good work friends overseas.

There was no knowing how people in Dominic's international professional world might respond to him if they did not have a context to help them understand what was going on. These friends offered to liaise with others if needed. The safety net expanded again, and together with Antony, who had a list of Dominic's international collaborators, these friends kept an eye on what was happening in Dominic's work world so I could get on with caring for him at home.

If Dominic didn't see the things from which he was restricted, he had a much better day; and he was easily distracted by the morning visits of friends. The cars were parked out of view in another street, the bicycles were in Felicity and Christian's garage, and I hid the car keys, office keys, and passports along with any alcohol, which Dominic could no longer self-regulate, in a locked cupboard. We hid the key to that cupboard in another room.

"Where is the key to the cupboard?" he would ask me, surprised by the fortifications denying him access to the places he had once been free to explore. "I need the car keys. I'm going to work."

He had worked out where his car keys were, but he couldn't work out the second step of how to find the key to the cupboard. I calmly said we would look for it, but would he like to go for a walk first? He usually said yes. I think I walked the whole of Brisbane and its surroundings. Closing the loop. Keeping him safe. Feeling the taste of deceit burn my throat like bile.

Summer was moving toward autumn. In Brisbane, there is no flutter of color before leaves fall, but the tropical thunderstorms disappear. I drove home from work in the cooler air and saw Dominic waiting for me on our treelined street, watching for my car. It was becoming harder to find activities that gave him a sense of purpose and his needs were beginning to demand more than it was fair to expect from friends. The Green Goblin had started to take up more space. I didn't know how much longer I would be able to work.

He saw me and waved, a smile stretching across his stiffening face.

I pulled into the driveway.

"Come, let's go," he said. He was ready to walk.

I went inside, put my bags down at the front door, and yelled hi to the boys. Then off we went. It gave them a break, and Dominic loved it. Dominic was talking less. I got to notice the trees, the changing color of the sky, and the sound of the birds. Hand in hand we walked. We walked and we walked.

When we got home, I started cooking dinner. I relied on a new batch of staple ingredients: 360-degree vision, the art of gentle distraction, and a great sense of humor. When I heard the call of our squeaky front door, I turned off the stove and left the half-chopped, half-cooked food to turn to rubber. I headed out to join Dominic, who was wobblier on his feet in the evenings, but still determined to wander down the street again. This would not be the only walk of the evening, but the boys were both working on assignments so I wouldn't ask them to finish preparing the meal tonight.

The hinge on the screen door called to us with the raucous squawk of a cockatoo multiple times a day as it opened and closed. It needed oiling, but it had become an inbuilt alarm, letting us know when Dominic had left the house.

"It's like a dripping tap," said Daniel on one of his visits. "How do you listen to that all day long?"

Unbeknown to me, Sister Patricia, a dear friend who had watched every step of Dominic's decline and was familiar with the squeaking screen door and my many street dashes, got on the phone to friends and arranged a meal roster. She soon had me covered seven days a week. Then she took a dementia course. Stepping in as my all-round guardian angel, adopted family member, and gatekeeper, she passed the lessons she learned there on to friends, helping them understand this particular disease and challenging the myths around dementia. I don't know what I would have done without her, my divine Sister of Mercy. You would never have known she was eighty-six years old. She still looks decades younger. She has more energy than most people half her age, sprays us with her wicked Irish humor, and enjoys a good glass of wine and a tot of after-dinner Bailey's. She is full of pioneering stories and has strong views on the rights of women. I think she is a bit of a rebel at heart, but her grounding influence is her kind and practical soul. She loves deeply and gives selflessly, but she's no pushover. She's totally connected to today's issues and nothing, absolutely nothing, shocks her. We have shared sacred secrets over the years, and she has seen life in a way that leaves her exceptionally wise.

The time had come to make more changes at home. Sister Patricia called me one afternoon. That morning, an occupational therapist had conducted a full assessment for home safety and suggested modifications that would enable Dominic to stay at home with us for as long as possible.

We needed shower rails, loo rails, and handheld showerheads; the shower doors removed; thermostat adjustment on our hot water system to prevent scalding; new easy-use kitchen taps; a higher bed and bed rails....The list continued. Eventually, we would need ramps.

Patricia invited me over for a cup of tea. Dominic was snoozing and both boys were at home. She lived a five-minute drive away and the kettle was on the go when I arrived. She pulled out two teacups as she chatted. She poured boiling water over the tea bags, added just the right amount of milk, and handed me a slice of homemade cake. The world is always softened by drinking tea made by someone else.

"Now, I have something for you," she said. "And don't get all proud on me. Just take it." She handed me an envelope with a very generous check. Someone had approached her and asked her to pass it on to me anonymously.

There must be a mistake. This was a big check. I looked at Patricia, speechless.

"People want to help."

The kindness of this unknown person reached down into the well of my sadness and had me bawling in relief. I had to stop working, but this money meant I would be able to get the house modifications done and buy some of the additional equipment Dominic needed. This was the first of many such gifts from a string of people, including family and friends overseas, whose unsolicited generosity continued to stun me.

Change and new things lay ahead for all of us. We were progressing backward and forward simultaneously. The boys and I drove to the university where Dominic had worked for Open Day. Nic wasn't sure of the courses he wanted to study when he graduated from high school, and we wandered around picking up pamphlets from various stands. Nic spent most of the time speaking with lecturers in the law and journalism faculties. I didn't think law was something he was particularly interested in, but when I saw the drop-dead gorgeous lecturer behind the stall, it all made sense. It was strange walking past the stand for Dominic's department and not seeing him there.

I watched a throng of eager young faces imagining the excitement of life on campus and independence away from their parents. For the boys, however, not having Dom there was a bit like having their membership to a family country club revoked. This was where they had hung out with him during school holidays when they were younger, making too much noise in his office, swimming at the pool, playing tennis, and meeting up for lunch in staff-only cafeterias. Displaced from dad land, they became invisible grievers. Would they still be able to go up into his department? they asked me. It had felt like their building, too.

We drove home with bags of information and no clearer idea of what direction Nic wanted to follow when he finished school. Nic was young for his year; he would graduate at sixteen.

"There's no rush to make big decisions now. Why don't you explore a bit by doing something more general and signing up for the courses you like?"

He shrugged.

"If you do what you like, you're more likely to end up somewhere you'll be happy."

"That's easy for you to say. Thing is—hey, there's Dad!"

Dominic was trudging down the middle of a usually busy street about 1.5 kilometers away from our house. Thankfully, we were the only car about, as he had no sense either of potential traffic or that he was in the middle of the road. I pulled over and walked toward him.

"Hi, this is a nice surprise!"

"There you are. I was coming to uni to find you."

"Where's Jo?"

No answer.

"Would you like to come for a drive?"

He smiled and climbed into the car. I called Jo, who had been at the house with him and was in a flat panic. I let him know Dom was with us. We drove around the block before making our way home.

Dominic was no longer able to determine the direction of sound. He was losing spatial awareness and depth perception. His physical reactions to the world around him had slowed. I read anything and everything to try and keep up with the Goblin. Journal articles, medical reference texts, books on the brain—anything I could get my hands on. The neurologist Oliver Sacks was my favorite. He talks about the function of judgment being one of the most important faculties we have. He says, "a judgment is intuitive, personal, comprehensive, and concrete—we 'see' how things stand in relation to one another and oneself." He goes on to say that people can get by without the capacity to form abstract or logical concepts, "but will speedily perish if deprived of judgment." Dominic was fast losing this ability. The doctors confirmed it. I made plans to stop work. Dominic was no longer safe alone. We continued to walk together. We walked and walked. Any effort to stop him increased his anxiety. If we just let him be, we could walk, hand in hand, into the quietness he was seeking, away from the demands and stimulation he could no longer manage.

Soon after Open Day, Dominic's position was advertised in the *Australian Higher Education Supplement*, but Antony had agreed that I could wait to pack up Dominic's office. Others would use the space, but nobody would touch *anything* until Dom had less awareness and I could do this without causing him any distress.

Michael dropped his backpack on the kitchen floor, opened the fridge, and started to drink fresh orange juice straight out of the bottle.

"Mike!"

He continued drinking. "Hey, guess what!"

"What?"

"I know this guy, Jackson, who is doing his first year in Dad's faculty."

In between glugs, he went on to tell us that his friend had come up to him that morning saying his lecturer had referred to a "Williams Theory" in class.

"That's your name—is this guy related to you?" Jackson had said.

Mike took him up a flight of stairs to Dominic's office and proudly pointed to the sign on the door: Dr. Dominic Williams.

"He's my dad," he said.

14

The doorbell rang and set off the wild wagging of Jessie's tail. She went to the door to sniff out who was there. We were a one-dog home now. Maxi had gone to live with Ed and Liz for a while, and the house was much quieter without her constant high-pitched yapping. She would come back to us later, but for now, Dominic couldn't tolerate the shrill sound of her barking reverberating inside his head like a wailing alarm.

It was 8:00 a.m. of my first day off work on indefinite extended leave—five months after receiving that bad-news phone call from Dr. Chen. My workplace was incredibly supportive. They offered me as much time off as I needed—no time frames, no expectations. They filled my position with locums, and said it would be there whenever I came back. At least I knew I had a job to go back to. I joined Jessie and opened the door to Felicity's smiling face and a warm batch of freshly baked raisin bran muffins.

"Are you okay?" she asked, taking in my daggy appearance. We talked as we walked to the kitchen.

"Dominic's not really sleeping at night."

"Do you need anything?"

"Mmm, a decent pair of pj's maybe?"

"pj's?!"

I started to laugh. Dominic was increasingly restless at night. The squeaky door would call out to me night after night, alerting me to his departure from the house. The previous night, when I woke to the squeaking door, I was wearing one of Dominic's comfy oversized T-shirts with holes under one arm and the nonmatching socks I had been sleeping in. I quickly slipped on an old pair of paint-splattered track pants before rushing out after him. It was some time past midnight. There was Dominic, gliding through the streets, with this tramplike woman with wild, knotted bed hair in hot pursuit. I could almost see the neighbors peeping through their blinds and hear them calling the police to report they had seen that disheveled vagabond chasing the poor disabled guy again!

Still holding the basket of muffins, Felicity started to laugh with me as I recounted my story.

"So, I'm thinking something a bit glam," I said. "If the police are going to pick me up, I might as well be arrested in style!"

Exhaustion was infused with humor and, laughing ourselves silly over a cup of tea, we imagined me dressed up in all sorts of arrest-worthy attire.

After finishing a second cup, Felicity washed the teacups, rinsed out the teapot, and made her way back to her home next door.

"We'll make dinner tonight," she called out as she left. I blew her a kiss from the front door and went back inside to get ready to take Dominic to another appointment. We were meeting with the geriatrician at the memory clinic, followed by a speech therapy session to assess Dominic's swallow. The ALS symptoms were fast encroaching. These appointments always left Dominic very tired. The walk back to the car became a slower shuffle; his breathing became raspy; increasingly he was more confused about where he was; and his eyes reflected the wordless anxiety of a man losing traction. It took so much effort for him to manage these appointments that, when it was time to leave, there was always less of him to bring home.

That evening Felicity and Disa arrived with a bottle of cold champagne. Jack and the boys were still next door making Italian and would bring it over when it was ready. Jack loves to cook. If his dreams of being an archaeologist don't work out, he could always become Australia's very own Jamie Oliver. Dominic was snoozing. Felicity poured me a glass and listened as I told her the latest details of Dominic's decline. The geriatrician had suggested I start looking into residential care options. I talked with the same frenzy as the bubbles fizzing their way up to the surface in my glass. Dominic was still a young man. The thought of placing my partner, my lover, my co-parent, my best friend in a nursing home tied my stomach in a knot so tight it prevented me from spewing up my distress. Dom was getting sicker, drifting away. How could we help him have a sense of his own story? How could we create for him a way of knowing and being known? How could we wrap him in it so he could *feel* it when he had no more words? How could we continue to remember him when none of our old Dominic was left?

"I'd love to make Dom a quilt—one he can take with him into care," I said.

"I'll help you," said Felicity.

"Really?"

"Really."

"Me, too; I love sewing," said Disa.

"But I'm not the greatest sewer; I'm not sure I'll manage some of that intricate quilt work," I said.

"You won't need to, we'll help. You can do some fabric painting. We'll sew that in, too. We can do anything really."

"Maybe we could incorporate some of the fabrics and scarves Dominic brought back for me from the different countries he traveled in."

"And let's add some African batik."

"And photos. Dominic often goes through our photo albums. Something happens when he looks at them, it's like he goes back there. You know the photos we have up all over the family room wall?"

Felicity and Disa nodded.

"He stands in front of them and touches them. I see his face change. He stops pacing and steps right into those worlds. Maybe he can choose photos that mean something to him, and I can transfer them onto fabric."

The evening unfolded with more champagne and hearty Italian food while the beginnings of Dominic's quilt plan were sketched out.

The center of the quilt would feature a large rectangular block, almost the length of the quilt, made up of our footprints—a different color each for Mike's, Nic's, Dominic's, and mine. We were walking this journey together. We would work the photos and hand-painted fabric blocks around this central piece and stitch in symbols with important associations for Dominic as the quilt evolved.

Michael and Nicolas started selecting images for the quilt that were significant to them.

"I want a photo of Dad and me playing."

"Let's use the trampoline ones."

"And the ones of him throwing us up in the air."

"Those are awesome."

"Yeah, they're *sick*!"

In these photos, the boys' young faces shone with adrenaline-filled laughter as they fell from outer space back into Dominic's arms.

As the quilt grew, these images were stitched together with more recent photos of each teenage son hugging a very sick dad, eyes closed, arms enfolding him as they absorbed the feel of him.

Painting Dominic's feet and getting him to walk across the calico laid out on the kitchen floor was another playful task. The fabric, spread out over several meters on the floor, made for a slippery surface. As I covered the soles of his feet with purple paint, he clutched the boys, standing one on either side of him to help him balance, and screeched with laughter. The brush and cold paint tickled. Soon we were all laughing, sloshing paint on each other like kids in a mud fight. I tried to stay in this playground and not glimpse the sadness that peeked between our toes as the boys and I pressed our colored footprints around Dominic's. Purple footprints danced across our kitchen floor for months afterward. We made no attempt to scrub them away.

As Dominic traipsed through the house on his pacing routes, we set up a workstation on our dining room table. Felicity is a master quilter, and she did as much sewing as possible where Dominic could watch and hear the chatter of stories being stitched together. In a way, he became the quilt director. Guided by his choices, I transferred photos to calico, and along with Felicity, Disa, and a few friends who joined us, we arranged and stitched them into each fabric block. Dominic made us endless cups of green vanilla tea, and as each square was completed, it was laid out on the table—a growing story on display.

There was something about the ritual of drinking tea that Dominic found comforting. It offered a mutual experience of being nourished by human connection without any expectations. There was no need for words. They were escaping him now, evaporating before the brew turned cold. In a conversation he was lost, but making tea for a friend offered him an opportunity to express some part of himself that was still linked, competent, and compassionate. He made it for everyone who visited, whether they liked it or not, and soon we learned to drink his carefully prepared offering poured from an unplugged kettle that had not yet been boiled. Green vanilla tea is quite good cold.

One morning, Dominic, the boys, and I were in the kitchen. I popped the kettle on and pulled out four mugs.

"Dom, how would you like your tea?" It was an automatic question.

I was thinking, *Sugar? Milk?*, anticipating an answer I already knew.

He looked at me in confused amazement as if I had just asked him the *most* ridiculous question known to humankind.

"In a cup."

Of course!

The boys and I started to laugh. Uncontrollable laughter grew from our bellies, inviting Dominic to join in. A contagious, collective laugh gathered momentum, rolling through the house.

"We should write a book about this!"

"We could call it *Green Vanilla Tea!*"

We chatted cheerfully or sewed quietly, adapting to when Dominic appeared vacant and working around his need to pace. We listened for the squeaky door above the hum of machines, and my regular street dashes became part of the quilt-making process.

"This photo is darling!" exclaimed Disa, leaning over Felicity's shoulder during one of these get-togethers. Five-year-old Dominic was smiling up at us from his Dominican Convent school photo. Jack and the boys were in the family room, transfixed in front of the PlayStation. Dominic was making tea.

"So, tell me," Disa asked over the buzzing sewing machine. "How did you and Dom meet?"

The first thing I noticed about Dominic was his eyes. He always said the first thing he noticed about me was my smile. Hard to avoid, really—I had braces at the time, a shiny mouthful of metal railway tracks. I was in the university cafeteria with a friend when he walked past in white shorts and a sky-blue T-shirt. His blond hair followed him in a curtained swish as he turned back to look at me. Our eyes met, and, right there and then, I knew.

I absolutely knew.

He walked backward, a little shy, still looking at me with those blue eyes. He tilted his head slightly to one side and self-consciously threw me a lopsided grin.

"I'm going to marry that guy," I said, nudging my girlfriend with my elbow.

She raised her eyebrows and looked at me sideways. "You don't even know him."

"I know."

I went home and, with unruffled certainty, casually announced to my dad, "I've just met the guy I'm going to marry."

"Oh yes? What's his name?"

I had absolutely no idea.

Over the next few weeks, I noticed Dominic in my psychology lecture. He always sat with the same girl in the center block, about one-quarter of the way down from the back. I was always with the same boy on the left of the lecture hall, just a couple of rows in front of him.

We both mistakenly assumed we were dating our class companions.

He told me later he used to sit a few rows behind so he could see me without being too obvious. One day, after a month of silently observing each other, I snuck out of the lecture. It was painfully boring, and I had an unfinished anthropology assignment due the next day. I didn't notice Dominic leaving the lecture hall until we bumped into each other in the foyer.

"Hi, Marie!" he said.

He knew my name? I listened to the sound of it float out on his breath and land on my shoulder. I blushed and he ruffled his hair. We acted nonchalant and threw around some small talk about the lecture being mind-numbingly dull.

"I saw you last week at the sports club with some of your gear. You fence?"

I nodded.

"Will you be there again tomorrow?"

"I think so."

"Me, too. See you there?"

"Okay."

"Yes?"

"Yes!"

I still didn't know his name.

Disa sat at the table, resting her chin in her cupped hands. "How old were you?"

I had only just turned nineteen.

Looking back at those stories and documenting them on pieces of fabric became a creative lifeboat when I was all at sea, but this quilt was so much more than a channel for my grief. Our conversations changed as the Green Goblin was given less airtime and, instead, we shared the stories of our life now being stitched together.

Double-bouncing Mike and Nic on the trampoline.

Singing "Nkosi Sikelel' iAfrika," the new South African anthem, and trying to teach the boys the words.

Snow fights and toboggan rides on Vancouver's Cypress Mountain.

Throwing two little toddlers sky-high, and catching them safely in big daddy arms.

Little boy giggles sprinkling themselves all over us.

Hearing the words, "I love you."

Capturing the simple yet poetic expressions of life. Catching them and sewing them into the quilt. Bridging the gap between memory and hope. Chaos had given birth to creativity, and the paradox became more familiar. I sat at the computer later that night, emailing my family between moments of Dominic's restless waking. Writing while sipping on hot tea, I watched the steam of Dominic's life linger above my cup before evaporating into the silence around me.

Somehow, even as we "lose" more of Dom every day, he offers us a new way to look at things. To be stripped of your past and to

*have no sense of your future leaves you firmly in the now. There
is no room here for attachments to the things we assume make us
happy. From my new world of shredded irrelevancies, there is no
mistaking what is important. Through Dominic's journey of dying
I am so much clearer about what brings life.*

The next morning, Dominic walked into the kitchen as Nic was
preparing breakfast: seven Weetabix and as much milk as the bowl
could take without spilling.

"Hey, Dad."

"Hey."

Nic opened his arms. Dominic walked into them. His shrinking
body nestled into the embrace of his growing son.

Dominic stepped back and looked at Nic's bowl with questioning
eyes.

"Like father, like son. You were the one who ordered two meals
for yourself when you took Mom out on a date!"

Dominic laughed. He walked over to the quilt table to look at
the new bits and pieces gathered there. Nic followed him with his
bowl of Weetabix.

"How many schools did you go to?" asked Nic, looking at the
different school badges and hatbands Dominic's mother had kept,
now stitched into the quilt. The family had moved a lot.

"Lots," said Dominic.

"Three, four…seven?"

"Lots."

Daniel tells a great school story of the Big Brother Legend. He
was twelve years old and Dominic, five years older, was in Year 12.

A schoolyard tough guy sauntered over and butted in to Daniel's
game of handball, bringing it to a standstill, knowing these little
tykes were too small and scared to respond with a slugfest. Then, just
in case they didn't know who was boss, he grabbed their tennis ball

and flung it across the playground. Unfortunately for him, big brother Dominic walked by. In a flash, this bullyboy was dangling in the air from his shirt collar, facing a ferocious tongue-lashing in front of the crowd before being dropped onto shaking knees. The boy never so much as frowned at Daniel again. Dominic the bully buster was Daniel's hero.

Nic moved his hand across to the square sitting next to the school badges. "This is such a cool painting—all our dogs and your dogs, too, when you were a kid." He read out the names: "Wellington, Brutus, Kita, Buster, Shep, Kim, Sasha, Maxi, and Jessie! I miss Sasha."

Dom smiled. Sasha had been our family dog in South Africa. Nic was a toddler when we left and has no real memories of South Africa other than our beloved Sasha. She was a lion of a dog, a huge golden mastiff who weighed fifty-eight kilos at only eighteen months old and carried not an ounce of fat. A gentler dog with children you could not imagine. Back then, little two-year-old Nic refused to go to sleep in his bed and insisted on sleeping with Sasha on her dog mat. She would lie on her side and lift her paw so he could snuggle up to her, and the two of them lay spooning until Nic fell asleep. She would lift her paw again when we came to take Nic, now slathered in dog drool, back to his bed. She would give herself a bit of a shake and readjust herself on her mat before drifting off to sleep for the night.

More stories like these joined the collection that spread across the dining room table. As friends came to visit, from academic colleagues to the boys' teenage buddies, they were usually welcomed at the door by Jessie and her wagging tail. The growing quilt gave us a different way to be with Dominic. It also gave Dominic a way to be with us. It didn't always soothe the shock of his obvious deterioration, but the boys were able to laugh with their friends about the dorky mullet haircut Dominic sported in his younger days, astounded that this could ever have been fashionable.

"Hey, I didn't know your dad played rugby! Dude, you play soccer—how come?"

"World's biggest sport, man—you can't beat that!"

"Do you know the words to this anthem?" The words of "Nkosi Sikelel' iAfrika" had been hand-stitched onto the fabric by a good friend.

"Yeah, but some of the words are hard to pronounce. You know it used to be banned—it was a liberation song during apartheid."

To the boys' mates, it was more familiar as the South African anthem sung at the start of rugby test matches, but before long, the boys would tell stories about Dom's and my involvement in social justice activities considered subversive back in the dark days of apartheid South Africa. Pets, sport, politics, family—so many contextual stories about us all that no one in Australia could possibly know. The rich yet invisible histories that accompany immigrant families on their journeys.

It was tough for any teenager visiting our home to know how to interact with Dominic. But the expanding quilt gave the boys' friends something upon which to anchor their conversations—an antidote to the awkwardness created by the Green Goblin.

Sometimes the pace of quilt making slowed. There were doctors' appointments, school activities, pacing, more doctors' appointments, washing of drenched sheets, endless loads of laundry, and ongoing midnight wandering. I slept in my running shorts and a T-shirt, with slip-on shoes ready under my bed. I would feel Dom get up and hope he would stay in the house. I kept an ear out in case he switched on the stove or boiled the kettle. He could not distinguish hot from cold. I had to watch that he didn't scald himself. When the door squeaked, I was up and out with him.

One morning, Felicity popped in with some of the blocks she had been working on at home. Dominic met her at the front door before she had a chance to knock. He said nothing, but the way he looked at her and reached out to touch the wedding square had her blinking back tears. They stood there until Dominic put his arms back by his sides again.

"They are yours," said Felicity as she handed them to him. Dominic smiled. He accepted the squares and walked over to the dining room table, adding them to the others on display. He laid them out and put his hand back on the wedding photo. He stood there quietly, tracing his fingers around the flowers in my hair.

I would often find Dominic spending time with the fabric photos, outlining the memories that gave him life. It took a few months to assemble the quilt top and insert padding for comfort and warmth.

We also stitched in a few blank blocks so that significant people could add to it by writing or drawing messages.

A few days after the quilt was finished, Genevieve rang.

"Hi, honey. Max is on his way over to help with the jammed sliding doors and the picture-hanging thing. He has Lilly with him. Is this a good time?"

"Thanks, yes, that's great."

"I'm out with Chloe now. Can I drop in tomorrow at about this time?"

"Tea will be ready!"

She laughed. "I have to find a way to get him to make me an English Breakfast tea." Green tea was not her thing. She hated the stuff.

Ten minutes after Genevieve called, Max, her husband, pulled up in the driveway. Dominic was in bed. Max knocked on the door holding a toolbox. Lilly stood beside him holding another of her pictures in both hands.

"This is for Dom," she said, before anyone said hello. She stood barefoot in a pink summer sundress. Her long ponytail, tied high up on her head, swished across her shoulders as she walked. She followed Max into our room, climbed up onto our bed, and sat next to

Dominic, cross-legged on a fresh set of sheets. She talked about her drawing with innocent comfort and moved in a little closer to show him the text she had added. She pointed to each word as she read out the message she had written. She smiled at him. Then she slipped off the bed and, with great concentration, her tongue peeping out the side of her mouth, she wrote her message on the quilt.

Diyar domanik, we wyll krawd you with au love.

Dear Dominic, we will crowd you with our love.

15

A few days after Lilly's visit, I heard a knock on the front door. Callie called out to me and let herself into the house at the same time. She had phoned the night before. I hadn't spoken to her in two years. I knew her, sort of, through a mutual friend. We had never socialized together. She had only just heard the news about Dominic. She had never been to my house before but walked herself through to the kitchen, accidentally knocking one of Lilly's drawings to the floor, and then started making herself at home, rummaging through the fridge and making herself a cup of coffee. I picked up the drawing and secured it back onto the fridge door with a magnet. She told me she had made cupcakes for us all and wanted to put them in one of our plastic containers. She said she knew I probably didn't have time to bake, and the boys would love them. They were chocolate cupcakes with chocolate icing and colorful sprinkles. She told me she remembered how much I loved chocolate. She would help with meals, too. What did we eat? Were there any allergies?

Dominic walked into the kitchen. He didn't know her. She looked him up and down as if he were on display in a museum.

"God, Marie, this is so tragic." She lowered her voice a bit. "To think of who he was before this..."

Dominic turned and left.

I stood there speechless, trying to untangle myself from what I had just heard. Dominic was smarter. He simply walked away and closed her out as he shut the bedroom door.

As Dominic's speech and comprehension became more compromised, a few Callies parachuted into our circle and assumed that because he didn't speak much, he couldn't understand anything. Sometimes they slipped into dementia speak, talking as if he were in preschool or in need of remedial education. Mostly, however, when people struggled, they spoke through him, as if he were invisible.

What was really interesting was how Dominic responded to them. For someone who was supposedly losing his ability to understand, he had them summed up way before we did. Somehow, whenever someone's desire to be part of his care was driven by a longing to meet his or her own needs, Dominic saw straight through it. Whether they were overzealous or anxious, he felt it and responded. He became an accurate barometer for any mood in the room.

Dominic's new emotional gauge had an uncanny way of picking up on our extraverbal cues. It compensated for his varying ability to import the meaning of words and his struggle to find the right words to express himself. He began to read emotional content with indisputable precision. He understood every nuance behind the words we spoke. He picked up the visual clues in our faces and could read the whole gamut of our unconsciously expressed gestures and behaviors. Dominic did not need words to grasp the meaning of interactions. I remembered my dream of Dom in the ice cube, unable to hear the words I spoke and watching the shape of me instead.

The week after Cupcake Callie had dropped by, Dominic and I went to a medical appointment. When we entered the consulting room together, the doctor greeted me and offered me a seat. Two chairs stood side by side against the wall. Dominic and I sat down and the doctor sat opposite us on a swivel chair in front of the examination table. He adjusted his reading glasses to sit lower on his nose.

Looking over them, he asked me a series of questions about Dominic, talking as if he were not in the room. Dominic was no longer a reliable historian, but it was a mistake to assume he had no way of understanding this environment and to behave as if he were not present.

. I turned to Dominic, communicating as much to the doctor as I was to him.

"Dom, is it okay if I answer these questions for you?"

He nodded.

"Will you let me know if I get anything wrong or leave anything out?"

Dominic slid his hand into mine.

The doctor swiveled his chair to face both of us. He continued to talk to me but at least he looked at Dominic. He softened, too, and for Dominic, there was no misunderstanding that. The rest of the appointment went off without a hitch. Dominic even laughed. He was relaxed and in good spirits when we drove home. I looked over at him from the driver's seat. He sat calmly and stared straight ahead.

Dominic started seeing a recreational therapist. The plan was to support him through an individually designed program that would engage him in purposeful activity and "enhance his emotional, physical, and social well-being." Dominic came home from the first session restless and intensely unhappy. He paced the kitchen, holding his head in his hands, back and forth, back and forth. He tried but couldn't describe to me what had happened. Then he showed me. He handed me a bath bomb—a cute, sky-blue ball of fizzy bath product—wrapped in transparent cellophane paper tied with a ribbon.

"You made this?"

He nodded, his face crumpled, crying without tears. He kept pacing.

Bath bombs? This is an intelligent young man, struggling with having lost a very successful academic career, and he's making bloody bath bombs?! How is this purposeful?

Never in Dominic's life had he been interested in crafts, let alone making pretty bath products. Why would now be any different?

Therapies like this focused on the storyline of Dominic's disappearance—they positioned him as a diminishing figure. They left no room for alternative stories that still thrived. They did not notice Dominic watching soccer games at school, where the family crowd knew the Dominic who loved watching both his kids play sport. He couldn't manage the noise of the basketball court anymore, nor a karate dojo, but he enjoyed the soccer field, where he could step away from noise and pace up and down. People were friendly; they tried not to stare. Brother Neil, the school principal, always made a point of coming over to say hello, never taking offense if Dominic looked straight through him or walked away halfway through a conversation. His language was kindness. He told me that Dominic reminded him of his best friend who had died of a brain tumor and behaved in very similar ways to Dominic. He, too, had lost a loved one to a green goblin.

The more I traveled in the company of this Green Goblin, the more I noticed the politics and power embedded in the ability to speak, the way various conversations shape our experiences, and the marginalization of knowledge that is wordless. Oliver Sacks says our natural speech does not consist of words alone. Instead, it "consists of *utterance*—an uttering-forth of one's whole meaning with one's whole being—the understanding of which involves infinitely more than mere word recognition." He goes on to say that language is immersed in tone and embedded in an expressiveness that transcends the verbal. He says it is deep, complex, and subtle, but perfectly preserved in people with aphasia (the total inability to speak). Not only is it preserved, he says, it is "preternaturally enhanced."

Such irony. For a man with no insight, the new, supersensitive Dominic could not only "read" people, but he could also feel the impact of his decline on them. Incongruence was not missed. If someone smiled through his or her anxiety, he would know. He felt that alarm. Anxiety would leap from that person's body into Dominic's. Because he was living in a body of wasting muscles, he found it harder to breathe when he was stressed. There is no denying that Dominic's decline was confronting and difficult to observe; that often we looked for signs, no matter how small, to indicate that dying might be getting better. Dominic had no way to understand this, nor could he soothe us, and any subconscious search for a sign of improvement in him was an inadvertent request from us that he make us feel better. He was never going to get better, and in order for him to be as comfortable as he could, we were the ones who had to manage ourselves.

As Dom interpreted his world in more adaptive ways, we learned to adapt with him. We had no checklist, and we made mistakes along the way. Dominic no longer understood abstract or metaphorical concepts. We no longer said things like "Geez, these mosquitoes are eating me alive!" We asked more yes or no questions so he didn't have to search for words. We watched for sensory overload; we spoke one at a time. We switched the TV off if the boys' music was on. We tried to be gentle and keep our tone calm. And we held on to laughter. When Dominic laughed at the woman on TV who turned orange and sparkled effervescently as she conquered the world after drinking Berocca, we laughed, too. We learned new ways to listen, new ways to speak, and new ways to see.

Importantly, the boys and I agreed to remind each other to take time out when we noticed the slightest glimpse of each other's frustration. Despite our love and patience, we knew with certainty there would be times when the Green Goblin would get the better of us.

One particularly grueling day, I heard Dominic ask Mike the same question a hundred times over. I tried every distraction to no avail, so I packed Mike off to spend some time at Jack's and took Dominic out for a long drive. Later, when I asked Mike how he was doing, he shrugged and said, "I try to forget with him, so I don't get frustrated when he asks me the same thing again."

Initially we suffered from new language fatigue, but, as with any language in which one is immersed, we soon became fluent. We learned not to challenge Dominic's thoughts, and we became better at noticing how he felt rather than arguing about facts. But it took us a while to get our heads around the driving conversation.

"Where are the keys? I'm going to the shops."

"But you can't drive."

"I can."

"No, the doctor said you can't."

"Of course I can."

Quiet panic. *What if this all goes downhill?*

Dominic had driven almost daily for half his life. He knew how to drive. Of course he could still drive.

Change of direction.

"Yes, I know you can drive. The doctor said you're just not allowed to drive at the moment."

"That's ridiculous."

"I know, it must be so frustrating."

"Ridiculous. I can't go anywhere."

"Where would you like to go?"

"For a walk."

And off we would go. Sometimes we would walk. Other times, if he wanted to go in the car, I'd take him for a drive.

Dominic was able to be with us in our sadness and in our joy.

He loved laughter and was drawn to kindness. Kindness can be shown without words. It echoes in the silence.

The key was to make peace with ourselves and to accept Dom exactly as he was. It called for an act of surrender. We had no bargaining power; the task was to live fully in the presence of dying. To open up another way of being, a way of gently reaching the soul and saying, "You are loved, you are safe."

As for Dominic, he never lost the skill of his implicit emotional knowing. It remained with him until the end. "The intelligence of dementia," the nursing home staff called it.

It would not be too long before Dominic would lie in a nursing home bed, resting in everyday confusion yet feeling the love of his best friend, Brian. I would read the emails he had sent to me to read to Dominic, written from his home in San Diego. How much of the content he understood, I don't really know. Dom could no longer read but each and every time I read one of these emails, his spirit came alive. In the first of these letters, Brian greeted him with the same affectionate banter they had always tossed around.

"Hello, you bastard!"

Dominic laughed.

Brian protested against the illness. He reminisced about the plans they had made to head off on adventurous kayaking trips together. He told Dominic that left without his kayaking buddy, he had taken up cycling. While out on his bike, he would keep looking around to see if Dominic was keeping up. He would try to ride by the beach as he knew this was Dominic's favorite place.

Brian chatted about Premier League Football and their favorite team, Manchester United. He kept Dominic updated with the latest scores and news about the Rugby World Cup coming up in France the next year. They had always agreed to back anyone who played rugby against England, but he was pushing it when he asked Dominic, a South African living in Australia, to join him as a Kiwi and support the All Blacks. Brian said how he missed him, and that no one could take away the crazy things they had done together. Maybe he would tell me about some of those things if Dominic didn't mind. He told him he loved him. Dominic heard it. He would bring his frail hands up from his sides and cross them over his heart. He would look at me through wide, unblinking eyes.

"Brian loves me!" With childlike glee, he would repeat himself. "Brian loves me!"

Brian was as good as right there with him, holding his dying friend in his arms, reliving kayaking adventures complete with their signature outdoor chess games along British Columbia's Howe Sound.

16

The trees in the Bunya Mountains soared up to the light. It was school holidays and, thanks to the generosity of friends, I was able to spend a week here with the boys. I took them away, hoping we could reach for some light of our own.

Our cozy mountain cabin was peacefully nestled in a rainforest national park. There were no shops close by, so we took our own food.

I packed our supplies together with old hiking memories: Dominic and me hiking with the boys strapped to our backs in child carriers through the Drakensberg; the four of us walking the forest trails in British Columbia; and our favorite, the trails along the Oregon Coast.

Before leaving the house, I went through to the boys' rooms and found one tiny bag of clothes that they had packed for themselves, buried under five supermarket bags of junk food. This was over and above the food I had already organized. It would be freezing, but even given the limited space in the car, there was no persuading them to exchange a bag or two of food for one of warm clothes. Not even the wildest imagination can grasp the appetites Mike and Nic had, or the quantity of food they were able to wolf down. There were many times I seriously considered changing their dinner plates for extra-large dog bowls.

Jack and Mitch came to this mountain cabin with us. These two best friends matched the boys plate for plate. I stood in the driveway, wondering how we were going to manage. The car was chockablock with food and luggage, and somehow we had to fold four long bodies in as well. What we really needed was a separate food trailer. Nic was right. Like father, like son: this need to eat must be a boy thing. Maybe a food story should go on the quilt, and a car story, too.

When we started dating, Dominic drove a 1960s VW Beetle—the type with a tiny nose protruding from the cover of the rear engine below the bug's small back window. I was nineteen, and I think the car was even older than me. His parents handed it down to him, and he drove it for years. It was our wedding car, too. This Beetle generated more noise than a construction site. One evening my little sister Reagen heard the roar of his engine and raced out to meet him at the front door of our family home. She was wearing a pair of my shoes, which were way too big for her eight-year-old feet.

"Hi," he said, ruffling her hair. "What are you up to?"

"Nothing." She shrugged, trying to look bored and hiding the childhood crush she had on him. "Where are you going?"

"Dinner at Fables—Marie reckons they have the best deep-fried eggplant."

"Eeew."

"That's what I think."

"No, it's heavenly, you'd love it," I said, walking in on the conversation.

"You can't love something that doesn't love you back," said Dominic.

"In this case, you can."

"It's horrible stuff," he said to Reagen.

Reagen clip-clopped to the verandah and stood on her tippy-toes to lean over the ledge and wave us goodbye.

"I think the muffler's broken," Dominic said as he started the engine. The car sounded like a tin of rattling rocks. The sky released a few ominous raindrops as Dominic reversed out of the driveway. Soon the rhythmic thudding of the windscreen wipers joined the cacophony of other car sounds as we made our way to the restaurant.

Just as we arrived, another somewhat battered student car pulled out of a parking spot in front of us. Dominic's luck with parking went back as long as I'd known him: spaces continued to free up for him wherever we were, no matter how busy the venue. Ushered in by the glow of a streetlamp filtering through the night rain, he pulled into the newly opened spot directly across the road from the restaurant. By now it was pelting down.

"Let's make a dash for it," I said.

"We'll get soaked."

"Let's try!" I said.

"Your smile—it's magic."

I blushed.

"You're blushing!"

"No, I'm not."

"Yes, you are!"

He was laughing now. He checked over his shoulder for traffic. The road was clear.

"Okay, here goes. One, two, three…"

The rain was warm and heavy, drumming loudly. I ran ahead, leaving Dominic to lock the car doors. When I reached cover, I combed my fingers through my long, wet hair, pulling it back off my face. I shook the water from my drenched cotton shirt, which now revealed the lacy trim of the camisole underneath. I was deliriously happy. If we weren't going in to eat, I would have stepped back out into the rain, open-armed and faceup, to feel it pour over me.

"I love this kind of rain! It doesn't keep you inside," I said as Dominic ran across the street to join me.

We made our way into the restaurant, my leather sandals squelching with every step. The place was abuzz with people, mostly lefty

Edmonton Public Library
Riverbend
Express Check #2

Customer ID: ************1298**

Items that you checked out

Title: Sarah's key
ID: 31221116371423
Due: May-16-18

Title:
 Green vanilla tea : one family's
 extraordinary journey of love, hope, and
 remembering
ID: 31221111582925
Due: May-16-18

Title: Psychology today
ID: 31221215042354
Due: May-16-18

Title: People
ID: 31221215090403
Due: May-16-18

Title: People
ID: 31221215062220
Due: May-16-18

Title: People
ID: 31221215045654
Due: May-16-18

Title: People
ID: 31221215052551
Due: May-16-18

Total items: 7
Account balance: $4.00
April-25-18
Checked out: 9
Overdue: 0
Hold requests: 1
Ready for pickup: 0

Thank you for visiting the Edmonton
Public Library

www.epl.ca

students and yuppies who, generally quite judgmental of each other, didn't seem to mind each other's company here. There were a few umbrellas dripping in the foyer, along with people waiting to be seated. There was a bit of a wait for bigger tables, but we were shown to our table for two straightaway. The restaurant had a trendy vibe; it was a well-known meeting place that did not break a student budget. A live musician belted out tunes on his guitar, competing with everyone's chatter as Dominic looked over the menu. I knew what I was having.

The server came back with complimentary garlic bread and took our order. Dom looked at me as if to say, *you go first*. I ordered the fried eggplant dish.

"It's popular tonight," said the waiter, scribbling down my order.

"I'll have the gourmet burger," said Dom. The waiter scribbled that down, too. "And the rump steak with extra mushroom sauce, please."

"Oh, do you have someone else joining you? I didn't realize you needed a table for three."

"No, it's okay, they're both for me."

"Oh! Like, did you want a starter? You've ordered two main meals. They are really big."

"The big meals will be great, thanks."

"Which one would you like me to bring out first?"

"I don't mind if you bring them out at the same time."

"You've got to be kidding!" I said when the server left. "You're going to eat all of that? He'll have a good story to tell in the kitchen!"

Dominic's teenage years saw him constantly ravenous, drinking liters of milk and eating fourteen slices of bread a day for high school lunches alone. This insatiable appetite never left him. When I joined his family for dinner, he would fill two dinner plates. One plate was piled high with rice and the other held the remainder of the meal, usually meat and an array of vegetables. Dominic didn't have an ounce of fat on him. Tall, athletic, and exceedingly fit, he ate more than I thought was humanly possible—until I had my own sons.

The wine arrived—a small carafe of the cheap house wine we could afford. Dom poured for both of us and lifted his glass, clinking it against mine.

"To the rain that doesn't stop you from going outside."

I kicked off my sodden sandals and popped my bare feet on top of his.

Without too much of a wait, a different server arrived at our table balancing two large plates up one arm and carrying a third in the other.

"The burger is for...?"

Dominic cleared a space.

"And the steak?"

"That's for me, too." Dominic moved the candle, the salt and pepper, and the carafe to one side, making room for the next plate.

"And the eggplant combo," she said, placing the dish in front of me. "Enjoy!"

"I think they pulled straws to see who could bring it out here. They want to see who the guy is that says he's going to eat all this!" I said.

Dominic smiled his crooked smile and opened up his burger, removing the beet with his fork.

"I'll have it. I *love* beets."

He reached over and added it to my plate. "You know, people throw the word love around without really thinking about the meaning."

"C'mon, the English language doesn't limit the use of words to one context. And you know exactly what I mean. The same word can have different meanings in different circumstances."

"I love my car. I love the beach. I love you. I love beets?"

I rolled my eyes at him.

"When it gets misused like that, it undermines the real meaning of the word."

"So you don't love the beach?"

"No. I really enjoy it, and I don't want to live without it, but I don't love it."

"And if someone is just being expressive and you know exactly what they mean?"

"Well, it bugs me. It's just used whenever to mean whatever."

A third server came up to the table and filled our water glasses. He stopped at a few tables on his way back to the kitchen, where I assumed the previous servers were waiting for an update on Dominic's progress.

We finished up, paid the bill, and left the restaurant. It was much quieter outside. The rain had stopped and a few playful stars appeared, glimmering in the sky like scattered glitter. Dominic put his arm around me. He kissed the top of my head as we crossed the road to his car.

My shoes still squelched.

Dominic turned the key, but the engine was dead—not a single splutter. "Oh well, here we go again," he said as he walked to the back of the car. "I'll push."

"Okay." I climbed over to the driver's seat, took off my soggy sandals, dropped them on the floor behind me, and turned the key. I depressed the clutch pedal with my bare foot, put the car into second gear, and took my other foot off the brake.

Dominic pushed.

"Now!" he yelled as we built up momentum.

I released the clutch, gave the accelerator a little push, and the car bunny-hopped back to life before the noisy engine exploded into sound. Dominic jumped into the passenger seat while the car was still moving. We laughed. We had become pros at this.

Our current Subaru Wagon was a lot more reliable. At least, now that we had kids, we had a car that worked. Dominic watched the boys pile their gear into the boot. It was sad to think he would never drive himself anywhere again. He would be staying at home with a carer during our time away in the Bunya Mountains. The carer was a nurse from a dementia-specific day respite center. A nurse friend at work had put me in touch with them. By now, Dominic had full-time care needs and we were struggling to get access to appropriate dementia support services for a young man who also had ALS, as well as for his family. Along with friends, we cared for Dominic with our limited options. At the time, there was no point of contact available to help me navigate the complexities of funding packages, home modifications, respite care, and at-home and residential care. There was no provider of age-appropriate support and information about what was available and how to access it. I case-managed it all myself until my nurse friend called on a few of her community resources and stepped in. I was fortunate; my work background gave me knowledge and some access to a system to which I was already indirectly connected.

Had I been an artist or documentary filmmaker—fantasies of mine—I might not have been as lucky. The day respite center looked after old people, but they were very good to us. They reduced the fees and provided us with some individualized respite care in our home, tailored around Dominic's younger-man needs and the needs of our family. They were supportive of me taking the boys away. However, they couldn't provide around-the-clock care, so during our time away in the Bunya Mountains, Ed helped out every day in the hours when the carer was not there. Ed had signed up for a degree at uni, and had an assignment due the next week. He had asked Dominic if he could use our place to work. He complained that his house was too busy with family activities to concentrate and write his assignments: the loud music, the kids' friends, the distraction— they took over the place. Dominic knew what this was like. Happy to help out his mate, he agreed, oblivious to the fact that he was being "looked after." Detailed lists were all prearranged—of emergency contacts, care needs, medication, modified meals, thickened fluids, daily routines, and spots where keys were hidden.

Ed stood with Dominic and me in the driveway, watching the boys trying to twist and fold themselves into the car. Once they were in, we were set to go. Jack was squeezed between Nic and Mitch in the backseat. His glorious curly, red, overgrown 'fro filled the rearview mirror and, while it didn't soften the guilt, it shielded me from seeing Dominic disappear from view as we drove away. The boys cranked up the music and, before we had reached the end of the street, I was driving a doof-doof car that propelled itself toward the mountains on the vibrations of Eminem's rapping.

We drove toward the Bunyas and into a completely different rhythm.

I emailed my family when we returned home.

The place pulsates with an ancient wisdom: deep, neutral, and life-giving. There's something about being out in nature. It's easier to listen when it speaks. Having come home, I can see how important it was for the boys to escape the intensity of daily life with a very sick dad. Away from it all, I noticed just how much they censor their everyday teenage life for him. They could be spontaneous, louder, more boisterous, less cautious, and less literal. They didn't have to hide things for safety and...and... There was laughter, hideous music, rainforest hikes, relaxing around the log fire, PlayStation, watching wallabies from the deck, and the view stretched to the end of the earth. For me it was both peaceful and very sad. Perhaps they sit naturally together somehow.

In the same email, I told them how Dom had no manic displays of behavior anymore. The parts of his brain that had once thrown up these wilder times had disintegrated. He remained emotionally blunted and was not usually able to initiate anything but, as we adapted to the changes in him, he had found touching ways to show connection. He was sweet and gentle. We held on to these times. But it made it harder to be mad.

We would still need to take breaks as, despite the greatest understanding, this new way of living was demanding, especially for teenage boys. Our trip to the Bunya Mountains had come on the heels of a family meltdown. Mike's and Nic's tolerance levels were shot, and frustration exploded out from under a worn cloak of patience. A yelling match had echoed through the house—wrestling, with slamming doors and language that would make a sailor cringe. No matter what I tried, I had no hope of dampening this fire. It was going to have to burn itself out. I took my frazzled self off to bed and lay there in tears. Dominic paced repetitively up and down from the bedroom to the study, dragging his hand along the wall now permanently decorated by a grubby smear. When he saw me go into our room, he followed. Unaware that he had been the cause of the blowup, he stood by the side of the bed. He leaned his stiffening body over mine, dribbling slightly, and lovingly stroked my hair. I closed my eyes, his touch recalling a time when the world was quieted under the stroke of his hands.

And then he was gone, back to pacing with his hand running along the wall.

The geriatrician fiddled with his pen during my next appointment with him. Dominic was deteriorating quickly. I had become accustomed to knowing that each doctor's visit would update me on the next set of bad news.

Dominic's gait, tone of voice, swallowing reflexes, and breathing all seemed to be changing, and his worsening cough spluttered through the night. He couldn't work the oven or stovetop, and if he tried, he was at risk of burning himself or setting something on fire. He needed help showering and dressing, and was unable to distinguish the hot tap from the cold. He ate cold food without feeling the need to warm it up, though he continued to generously make our guests cups of green vanilla tea.

I wasn't always sure which symptoms to attribute to dementia or to ALS as Dominic's body progressively shut down, shedding functions.

It cannot be easy living in an unreliable body with a scrambled brain and debilitating confusion. One week after my appointment with the geriatrician, I took Dominic to the hospital for a swallow X-ray and more breathing tests. Here Dominic encountered escalators that did not wait for his legs, the swish of busy people with places to go, beeping machines that drowned out the reassurance of my voice, buzzers joining the squeaks of wheelchairs, and the sound of his name being called from unknown faces. His sensory system was completely overloaded before the tests even took place.

Hospitals were no longer places he could manage.

On our way out, I avoided the escalator and took the elevator down to the ground floor. The automatic doors slid open for us as we approached the main entrance. We left the building and walked out into a sunny afternoon. Suddenly, Dominic's hand left mine and, with an agitated turn, he dashed into the traffic. He didn't hear my calls. Disoriented and confused, he paced unpredictably in the middle of the road with cars coming from both directions. He weaved in and out, clasping his exploding head in both hands, trying to switch it all off. I waved my arms at the cars to signal them to stop and stepped out into the traffic after him. The bewildered drivers watched as I took Dominic's hand.

"Dom, it's me."

"Marie...Marie..."

"I'm here. I'm right here."

I squeezed his hand. "Let's go home." I put my arm around him and led him back to the pavement, hoping we would make it safely back to the car.

Later, in the middle of the night, I found Dominic standing quietly looking at the quilt. He was restless and couldn't sleep. I noticed he was holding a framed photo of the two of us, wrapped in each other's arms, laughing, with no sense of what was to come. He looked from the frame to the same photo that had been transferred onto the quilt.

The night was quiet.

"I feel angels around me," he said. Dominic spoke of this often.

I smiled—there was something comforting about this for both of us.

He turned to look at me.

"You are one of them," he said.

He saw me tear up.

"It's true. You are an angel to me."

Unexpectedly lucid, he took the photo back to bed with him. He lay down and kissed it. He placed the photo on his chest, holding it with both hands. As he relaxed toward sleep, he handed me the frame.

"I love you," he said.

"I love you, too."

"Please..." He pointed stiffly at the dresser. "I want to see it when I wake up."

I placed the picture on the dresser and climbed into bed with him.

"I'm not getting better," he said.

I held him. His words started to disappear again, but when I asked what he needed from me, the words he found said everything.

"Just be nice to me."

17

I always knew nursing home placement was what awaited us. Doctors had mentioned it several times, but I held it far away in the distance until events forced it into closer view. This time it was in writing. The geriatrician wrote on Dominic's latest report: "It is likely that over the next few months he will require placement in a nursing home..."

There were no facilities available for young people. A new not-for-profit organization, Youngcare, was getting a lot of press, but its residential facility was not yet built. If we were ever unable to care for Dominic at home, placement in an aged-care facility was our only option. I was going to have to start looking for suitable places.

Beth came over and took Dom for a drive so that I could go out to "do my research." She drove out to Bribie Island. She realized she had been driving along the Bruce Highway for ages and wondered out loud if she'd missed the turnoff.

"Yes," said Dom. "You did. It was back there." He didn't flinch.

In the meantime, I hopped in my own car to collect Sister Patricia. She had insisted on coming with me to look at potential nursing homes. The plan was to have coffee together, somewhere nice, between each visit.

I was calm and quite unfazed about the day. It was all rather academic, really. I was simply checking out the possibilities in advance so that if this ever had to happen, I would not have to make any big decisions in a crisis. Given the waiting lists, I wanted to have the advantage of time to develop relationships with people rather than being some unknown name on a list.

The first stop was not far from home. It was a beautiful building from the outside. We were a bit sneaky with this visit. We deliberately did not make an appointment, but went to visit one of Patricia's friends who lived there. She made us tea and we chatted about what life in the nursing home was like. She was ninety years old, an immaculately dressed woman who took great care with her appearance. She greeted me with a smile and stroked her soft wrinkled hands over her neatly set hair. She showed me two of her new dresses and I had to agree that the wardrobes provided were way too small for her collection of clothes. She reached for her walking stick and took me on a tour.

"Darling, I think it would be hard for anyone young to live here." She walked me past a room where a thirty-something, severely brain-injured woman lay.

"Car accident, I think. This poor thing gets no visitors, but the nurses are always cheerful."

She walked on, leaning heavily on her stick.

"Your Dominic, can he still walk?"

"Yes."

"I'm so sorry you have to be doing this, love."

"Thank you."

"They put people that wander downstairs, you know. I can take you there."

"Is it a secure ward?"

"Yes. We can get in but they can't get out."

We approached a set of wooden stairs with beautiful banisters, smoothed down by the wearing of hands over time.

"Is there a lift we can use?"

"Yes, but we're fine," said Patricia and her friend. They held on to the rails and slowly made their way down.

Despite the attractive trimmings, I felt as though we were descending into dungeons tucked away from the rest of life. Patricia's friend pushed on the ornate wooden door at the bottom of the stairs. I wondered what it screened. The first thing to reach me was the smell. The place reeked of disinfectant. I stepped into a bare central living room area with shiny floors crisscrossed with the scuff-marks of wheelchairs. Men and women sat in their wheelchairs lined up against the walls. Slumped over with chins buried in their chests, they looked like ragdolls hanging motionless from hooks on the wall. The three of us stood in a room devoid of life.

A loud, jovial nurse was talking in the adjoining dining room. She got up from her seat at one of the tables and offered to show me around.

I asked a few friendly questions and then she had to leave me to tend to a new resident who was banging on the door trying to leave the locked ward.

Patricia looked worried, but I left there in good spirits. It was simple. Dominic was not going there, even if my life depended on it. Michael and Nicolas would never see their dad in a ward like this. We said our goodbyes. I thanked Patricia's friend, and Patricia and I went out for our coffee.

The coffee shop was nestled in a gift shop cum florist's. We sat in a shady spot outside on the patio, surrounded by flowers sitting in buckets of water and a jasmine vine climbing over the fence. Its shiny leaves looked as if they had all just been polished. The small, white, star-shaped flowers would release their fragrance into the air in the evening, just like the plant at home on our deck. Dominic loved sitting there. It was one of the few places he could sit still for short periods of time.

Our coffees arrived. I couldn't help thinking about Dominic and how his drinks now had to be thickened. He hated thickened tea.

There was so much life in the simple act of drinking tea. Not to be able to sip on it seemed unfair. He needed full supervision with all of his meals, as he was at risk of choking. He was aspirating, but he wanted his regular cup of tea.

Patricia scooped the froth from her cappuccino with a teaspoon.

She was good with silence. I stirred my coffee, swirling my thoughts around the mug in circles. There were other things to consider alongside whether or not to thicken drinks. Earlier that morning, Dominic had been out on the deck with me. The birds were still singing their welcome to the day. He disappeared for a while. I knew he hadn't left the house, as I hadn't heard the squeaky door. I went inside, walked to our bedroom, and noticed the door leading into our bathroom was closed.

"You okay, Dom?"

No answer.

"Can I come in?"

"Yes."

I opened the door. Dominic was on all fours, kneeling in shit pooled across the floor. He was scooping up the accidental spill with his bare hands, trying to clean up, but bewildered and not sure what to do.

"Can I help?"

He nodded. I closed the door behind me and squatted down on the floor with him.

"You okay?"

He nodded again with a small smile of embarrassed confusion, and when he sensed I didn't seem at all fussed by the whole thing he relaxed. Using wads of toilet paper, I scooped up some of the mess and dropped it in the toilet. I threw a towel over what was left. I reached for his hands and, with a wet cloth, gently wiped away the warm smears of his body's betrayal.

As I stood up to run the shower, he reached over and tried to put his soiled shorts back on.

"I'll get you a clean pair."

"No!" He tightened his grip on the waistband, determined to put this particular pair back on.

"Okay, but how about a shower first?"

He released the shorts and allowed me to take off his T-shirt. He held on to me for balance and then took my hand, stepped into the shower, and let the warm, soapy water wash him clean. He showed no signs of distress. On his own cue, he came out of the shower and, still wet, tried again to dress himself in his soiled shorts. I wasn't quick enough! *I should have hidden them.* I tried to distract him.

"No! My shorts!"

He needed another shower. *Please let this work.* He followed my prompts, stepped back in under the water, held on to the handrails and let me wash him again. I squirted him playfully with the shower nozzle; he laughed. I was slowly getting very wet. I reached down and slid his shorts under another towel where he couldn't see them.

"Just enjoy the warm water for a sec."

I made a quick, wet dash into the bedroom to get a clean pair.

"My shorts!"

Unbeknown to Dom, I had bought six identical pairs of blue shorts. They were easily washable and did not need ironing. They had an elasticized waist so that he did not have to struggle with zips and buttons. The incontinence pads were discreetly hidden and nothing was noticeably different with his T-shirts hanging loose like he had always worn them. He still looked like Dominic—kind of beachy and casual, pretty cool.

"Here they are." I held up a clean pair.

He smiled. Every pair looked like the ones he had been wearing. He started to shiver. I turned off the water and wrapped a fresh towel around him. Before I could redirect him, he stepped onto the towel that had soaked up his insides and walked away without noticing the soiled footprints that followed him across the bedroom carpet.

I told Patricia this story. She reached over the table and held my hand.

"You know McCorely Nursing Home?" she said.

"The place we're going to visit next?"

She nodded. "They would support you in all this, you know. You wouldn't be alone there."

My silence said more than I realized.

"I know. We're just looking." She finished her coffee. "I don't want to go into care either, and I'm old."

McCorely was a fair drive away, fifty minutes or so. Many of Patricia's Sister of Mercy friends lived there as residents. These women had all entered the convent together as young novitiates. Many of them had joined in Ireland before coming out to Australia. Somehow, under the leadership of their founder, they had managed to be self-regulatory rather than fall under the direction of bishops. Seems this was an order of pioneering women, "walking nuns" who, right from their beginnings, worked out in the community. Whether Patricia and her friends had worked in social justice, poverty, education, or care for the sick, they had lived much of their lives together in religious communities, and now they were entering aged care together. This would have to be better than entering a facility not knowing a soul, leaving shared lives and friendships behind, and having one's last days reduced to four walls and a window. McCorely Nursing Home had recently opened its doors to laypeople. I wondered what it was like for them to have others join them.

We parked the car on a grass verge under the dappled shade of gum trees. When I walked through the automatic doors of the nursing home, the reality of Dominic's impending placement churned through me like wet cement. And yet there were times I longed for the relief it might bring. Oh, the guilt of thinking such a thing! My conflicting emotions fought it out in a screaming headache that would not go away.

Two of Patricia's friends were sitting in the lobby. She greeted them. They smiled at me and greeted me by name.

No! I do not want to fit in here!

I smiled politely. I imagined a lot of the nuns here continued to live out their vocations, caring for each other and their coresidents, but I did wonder if there were any sadistic, psychotic ones hiding among them, roaming the McCorely corridors with steel rulers. If Dominic bumped into the likes of Sister Eusebius, the nun who beat him in primary school, things could get really interesting.

I looked beyond the two women, through the glass doors and over the large grounds with landscaped gardens. The way the bougainvillea fell reminded me of my old school friend's garden in Durban. Sindy had called me just a few days before from South Africa. I missed her. We had lovely wedding photos taken in her garden. The woody vine filled with papery red blossoms had stretched its arms over Dom and me in a natural arch. After six years together, we were still young, with a lifetime of shared possibilities ahead. We were married in a small, relaxed wedding in Dominic's school chapel followed by a garden lunch at Sindy's place.

I had spent the night with her before the big day. The plan was to have some girlfriend time together, but I was so nauseous with morning sickness that she spent most of the time making me black tea and hoping I would not spew during the ceremony the following day.

Dominic arrived the next morning to pick me up. I opened the front door barefoot, wearing a long cotton dress and flowers in my hair.

"You look beautiful," he said.

I threw my arms around him. "I smell petrol!"

"You can still smell it? Have you got any mouthwash?"

"What happened?"

"The Beetle ran out of petrol so I had to siphon some and then I had to push start the car. I didn't even know if I would have enough to get here!"

"You're kidding."

"No, we have to fill up on the way to the chapel…"

I started to laugh uncontrollably.

Dominic had another quick shower, after which Sindy and her mum offered to drive us to the chapel in their Mercedes Benz. No pressure. What did we think? Would we consider it? It might be a good idea. What if we didn't make it to the petrol station?

Dominic and I would sooner break down in our dilapidated Beetle than submit to a ride in a car that symbolized bourgeois life. We declined. I only hope we did it graciously, but I suspect we did not. Sindy and her mum were very patient. They showed not an ounce of frustration toward these two young idealists, and it was agreed we would give the Beetle a go. I threw my shoes in the back, seat, lifted my dress up onto my lap, and sat in the passenger seat. I placed my two bare feet on either side of the hole that had rusted through the floor, exposing the road beneath it. Sindy and her mum followed us to the service station in case we ran out of petrol again before we got there. We filled up the tank and made our way to the chapel in our noisy Beetle, decorated with blue wedding ribbon, followed by a shiny black Benz, our backup car.

I did not spew. The day was all happiness and sunshine. Sun shone through stained glass windows on promises of love. The light in each other's eyes. This man of loveliness; the man of my everyness. I woke the next morning feeling the warmth of his sleeping breath on my skin and the protection of his hand resting on my naked, swelling belly.

The sound of a wheelchair reoriented my body to the nursing home lobby. I noticed a wooden carving on the wall. In it I saw the image of a tree—a eucalyptus tree, I think. The leaves were draping down and through them I saw children playing, little cottages, and an old person with a walking stick. It was a hand-carved story of some kind, a story about the Sisters of Mercy on this site. Their roots. Stories of things accomplished, things celebrated, things that would be remembered. I ran my hands over the wood, my fingers following the carved lines of time that opened out into each other.

A tall blonde woman walked toward me. She wasn't dressed like a nurse, and her shoes made a clip-clop sound when she walked. In the months to come, I would listen for that sound in the corridors. It would add the pulse of kindness into the rhythm of dying. She welcomed me and warmly introduced herself. Her name was Maggie; she was the Director of Care. I liked that—a Director of Care, not a Director of Nursing. I liked that a lot. I spent some time with Maggie and another key member of staff that morning. I checked out their model of care, their credentials, their care philosophy, their values, their staffing ratios, their dementia-specific care, their attitude toward and connection with families, their ideas about caring for a young man when they were geared toward nursing the elderly, their palliative care, their everything care—no stone left unturned. They sat patiently through the "Marie test," letting me fill the room with all my vulnerabilities. I was taken with their integrated model of dementia care. No one here was locked up. They showed me around and poured me endless cups of tea, but offered no pity. I was so relieved. Pity can be very isolating; there is nowhere to go from pity. One remains locked up in a sad story, alone. Pity has a way of creating and preserving hierarchical relationships between people that by their very structure assume that the positions and abilities of the pitied are "less than." It has nothing of the warmth and reciprocal human connection that comes with compassion.

I told our story. The plight of our young family touched them and, to my great relief, they did not seem to think I was a bad person for considering placement. They held our story with a balance of authentic empathy and professional competence, and they were kind—a tangible kindness that changes things and stays with you.

At the end of the visit, Patricia and I walked across the road to my car. She put her arm around me. We sat quietly in the brokenness before driving home.

A beef stroganoff was sitting on our kitchen counter when I got home.

It was still warm and covered in foil. Next to it were a bunch of brightly colored gerbera daisies and a note from my good friend Bea, who lived just up the road.

> *Taking you to Ladysmith Black Mambazo next Friday, got tickets already. Be ready at 7:00 p.m.! Love, B XOX*

Our freezer was packed with meals, and people were now dropping off warm meals, freshly made that day. Sometimes they added a bottle of wine, a card with kind words, or a magazine I wouldn't have time to read. Streams of rostered meals arrived, prepared for us by friends and friends of friends: people I did not even know. Between them the ironing was done, the lawn mowed, and the house cleaned. We were nourished by support that remained overwhelmingly generous. I had no idea so many people cared about us. I was so fortunate to have all this wonderful help. I could not manage without it. The downside was that our home, which had once been a sanctuary, now felt more like a transit station.

Nights were filled with a different kind of busy. Our nighttime street wanders continued. Dominic took to wanting breakfast anytime between 3:00 a.m. and 5:00 a.m. Given his difficulty swallowing and general problems with safety in the kitchen, I needed to be awake whenever he was. His cereal needed to be mushy to help him avoid choking on it, but the bigger trick was trying to get through these early morning breakfasts without waking the whole household, especially during exam time. All the lights would go on, dishes would clang, and cupboard doors would slam as he looked for things. Pacing between spoonfuls of soggy Weetabix, he would repeatedly try to pop into the boys' rooms, wanting to know who should be woken up for school.

"C'mon, get up, you have to go to school."

"Daaad! It's the middle of the night."

"You'll be late."

"Okay, thanks," they would say, and turn over.

I remembered the years before the Green Goblin came to stay, when the boys would do anything to avoid getting out of bed in the mornings. Dominic would go in and wake them for school.

"First, he'd switch the lights on without any warning," said Nic when we were remembering these earlier times. The boys would grunt and put their heads under their pillows.

"Then, he'd prance exuberantly toward the bed, laughing unsympathetically at my attempts to block him out." Nic would continue to lie there, motionless. The battle of wills was on.

"Next, Dad would whip the bed covers off in one fell swoop. It was a killer in winter. I'd lie there shivering, determined to ignore him. Then he'd grab my ankles and start pulling me off the bed, singing that stupid 'good morning, isn't it a lovely day, I'm so glad I'm going to school today' song in an overly happy voice."

Before long, this would turn into the predictable ritual of rough-and-tumble before school as whichever son was being dragged out of bed would hold on to bedposts, refusing to be defeated, until eventually they were on the floor wrestling with enough energy to kick-start their day.

Perhaps some part of Dominic remembered these fun times. Most often I was able to distract him away from their doors, but then Jessie's sleepy face would inevitably brighten up. She'd wag her tail, thinking it was time to play, barking with Josh Groban on the stereo that Dominic had cranked up to welcome the house into midnight song.

Chaos, peace, chaos—I was getting better at navigating it. Nocturnal Weetabix adventures became a regular occurrence. I disconnected the stereo in the family room and used a portable one.

Most often Dominic followed the music, and me, back to the bedroom, where he let Josh sing him back to sleep.

Chaos, reprieve, chaos. The Green Goblin had a way of inviting, and sometimes escorting, us back to its oppressive cell of restrictions. I kept the music in my ears, but the bars were always there. I had to decide on which side of the bars to stand. I wrote to my dad.

Dominic was doing better for a couple of weeks but it looks as though things are starting to change again. I was at an appointment today. Weird how your head can be ready for inevitable changes, but never your heart. I don't want Dom to suffer and I don't want to say goodbye. With each new step, this journey is filled with more paradoxes: my greatest wish is also my greatest fear. What I wish for is what I don't want.

Genevieve left her family of five kids at home with Max and stayed overnight at our place once a week to nurse Dom. She insisted I try to get some sleep. I was beyond tired. She is a registered nurse, and Dom really liked her. I would force myself to walk past the mounting home administration that needed to be done, make my way up the road to Bea's house, and sleep there. If I stayed at home, an anxious Dominic would come looking for me. In-home respite provided me no reprieve if I was still in the house. A couple of friends took Dominic out of the house for drives; a work colleague coordinated the aged-care assessment process required for both home-care funding packages and high-care nursing home placement; and, through this, we were finally able to expand the in-home respite care hours a little. I used these hours to go to the boys' sports events on the weekends, their after-school events, and other things, like parent-teacher interviews.

One Saturday afternoon, I was at school watching Nic's soccer match. Soccer never drew the huge crowds that rugby did, but they had quite a lot of support that day. Nic's team was playing a rival school they had to beat—their pride depended on it. Brother Neil came over, as he did every weekend, to say hello and check in.

"Don't worry about the school fees. We have them covered."

I stared at him in disbelief. There was a roar from the crowd. Someone had scored a goal and, from the sound, it was our team. In amongst the noise, I vowed to pay them back, and thanked him profusely, but how do you find adequate words of thanks at times like that?

"No, it is the other way around," he said with a smile. "This is *our* thank-you to Dominic for the gift of his two sons." He put his arm around me before leaving to join the crowd. "And it is our pleasure."

I heard another roar from the field. A teacher, also the school photographer, was on the sideline, taking pictures of the game. When Dominic had been well enough to join us, this same man had asked Nic if he could take pictures of Dominic watching his games. He took some lovely photographs of a very sick dad proudly supporting his son's soccer matches. We added one of them to the quilt, which made a visit to school some weeks later. The boys were happy for a few teachers who had closely supported them to see it, and hoped they might contribute a message or a simple signature.

What a great human being to inspire such love and to be a father to such wonderful sons.

Sharing a little of the journey of the Williams family and meeting Michael and Nicolas shows just what a privilege it is to teach. Thank you, Dominic and Marie. Peace and blessings.

As the teachers added their messages, one of them stroked his hand over a hand-drawn picture of four trees.

"Can you tell us about this one?"

Next to the drawing was a tribute written in green.

4 trees
4 lives
Dominic, your love will grow with us forever

Simon and Molly had drawn this message. They had planted a garden that they wanted Dominic to enjoy before he went into care.

Dominic had watched Simon and Molly digging up our garden while he sipped at his tea, without understanding the significance of what he was watching. With each thud, their shovels dug deeper, opening up the earth that would feed four new trees.

When the planting was done, we sat around the patio table enjoying a fresh pot of tea. Dominic was stooped, his eyes vacant, unaware of the drool that made its way slowly down the side of his open mouth. Nic left the table and went through to the study. I could see him through the window. He was crying—his shoulders hunched over as his arms cradled his head. I got up to go to him.

"Let me do it," said Simon.

Through the window, I saw Simon enter the room and take Nic in his arms. Without saying a word, he cried openly with him.

Before Simon left that afternoon, he wrote the boys a note.

The Four Trees

We planted four trees. These trees represent the Williams family and the life that lies ahead. Three of the trees are planted together; these trees are for Marie, Michael, and Nicolas, planted together for security to share the earth and the energy and life force it has. These trees are from South Africa. They are tough and hardy, can survive any conditions, and will grow into strong, big trees, just as you will grow and mature.

The single tree planted apart is for Dominic as he leaves you and continues his journey. He will, as the tree, grow and flourish and develop into a magnificent flowering tree....One day, Dominic will be gone but the lone tree and your trees will stand strong and beautiful. They will carry on growing. I will miss your father but I can at least plant a tree for him. Dominic's tree is from Sri Lanka, one of his favorite spots.

Love, Simon

18

The phone rang.

"Who is it?" I mouthed at Mike.

He shrugged as he handed me the receiver.

It was Maggie, letting me know that a respite bed had become available. There had been no vacancies for the next eighteen months but someone had cancelled, which would free up the dates over the boys' end-of-year exams—in fact, the exact dates of Nic's final Year 12 exams and all the end-of-year graduation ceremonies. The timing was uncanny. They didn't want to stay with friends, and I didn't want the same nightmare at home as Mike had been through the previous year for his Year 12 exams. The geriatrician's last conversation with me a few days earlier rang through my head. I looked over at Patricia, who was sitting on our patio.

"Take it," she said, quite matter-of-fact. "You can always cancel it later."

I accepted, put the phone down, and stood there. *I can always cancel later. It's not a permanent thing, it's not a permanent thing.* But I knew. Dominic would not come home.

The geriatrician had referred us to another doctor, someone who could help Dom with the next stage. I sat in his windowless office, hearing myself talk about end-of-life issues: requests for nonresuscitation; no PEG feeds (percutaneous endoscopic gastrostomy, a procedure used to insert a feeding tube into the stomach through the abdominal wall); no invasive interventions; and when to hold back treatment for aspiration pneumonia, a much grayer area. Dom and I had talked about these things years ago, when life was strong and full of promise, hoping we would never have to enact them and trusting that, if ever it were called for, we would do what was needed. The part of me that hovered above myself and wasn't participating in this conversation noticed how bland the walls were—pale gray-blue, like dead skin. The part of me that was earthed heard the clarity of every single word.

One week later, the third of October, was our wedding anniversary.

I went into the clinic and met with the new specialist. She was kind and frank. Four to six months, she thought, if that. She told me what to expect. We had the same end-of-life conversations again. No prolonging anything, no holding on to life. Making all this kinder. Gently letting go. Palliation is very different from the world of diagnosis and treatment. It is softer and closer. And so much sharper.

Back at home, Dominic was lying down, and the phone rang again. After the call I sat at the computer, my world swirling, and wrote. Writing slowed the world down. The space between writing and pressing the send button gave me time to pause. I could linger there trying to capture my thoughts, the essence of which may have vanished in a conversation.

I wrote so that the part of me that didn't know what to do would be held by my family when they woke up to their morning.

I worry about the boys—how do I lessen the impact of something like this for them during their final exams? The palliative doctor was kind and we looked at options. She'll try to manage Dominic's symptoms over the next six to eight weeks to get us through the exam period, but there will be no invasive interventions. We'll continue, with great love, to provide Dom with dignity, comfort, and help to manage any pain. I'm not sure how much to say to the boys right now. We've always been so open and honest, but Michael is in the middle of exams. It's such terrible timing. Things are taking a toll. They are exceptionally patient with Dominic, but the strain in all of us is showing up in other ways. It sort of turns things on their side, or on their head, maybe even inside-out. And then, somehow, in the middle of all the upside-downness, the boys show me their wisdom.

I wrote on about a mother of one of Nic's friends who had called a few days earlier, saying some of the boys at school were worried because he wasn't talking about "things."

"It bugs me," Nic had said when I asked him about it. He lay on his stomach, stretched across his bed, while Mike chewed on a mint and leaned his tall body against Nic's bedroom doorframe. I moved Nic's smelly sports bag aside and got comfortable on the floor. He turned onto his side, propping himself up on his elbow. Mike threw him a mint.

He raised his arm and caught it without taking his eyes off me.

"People say I never talk about it." He put the mint in his mouth. "But I don't want to talk to all of them just so that they can feel better that I'm talking. Talking with them doesn't change anything."

"I agree," said Mike. "There's no relief. It's like not being able to wake up from a nightmare."

"And then, when they keep asking you and nothing's changed, or things are worse—which they're gonna be—you have to talk about the same nightmare over and over again. They feel better 'cause I've talked, and I feel like shit!"

"We'll talk to someone if we want to."

There is one certainty in all of this—things will get worse. Today has been a weird serendipitous day, taking us one day closer to it all. This morning, before seeing the palliative doctor, the center that provides in-home help for Dominic told me his needs are more than they can manage now. They advised me to consider nursing home care. Coming from them this was a shock, as they very much believe in community care. When I told the doctor about Dominic's possible respite stay, she strongly encouraged me to place Dominic permanently if I could. Then, just as I got home, Maggie rang...

Maggie's call had surprised me. Life tumbled through the everyday circus acts of dementia and I was "on duty" twenty-four hours a day, seven days a week. I was so tired that I could hardly see straight, but when Maggie called from the nursing home and asked if I would be ready to accept the bed as a permanent placement rather than respite, I dissolved into tears.

"Permanent?"

"What are your thoughts?"

"I don't know...I'm just so tired..." *How do you stop weariness from becoming ugly, graceless?* "I want to be able to keep on loving him."

"We can help you to do that, to keep on loving him. You'll be able to rest. You'll have access to so much more of each other then."

"Do I have to decide right now?"

"No, it's okay. Why don't you come in for respite as planned?"

I silently thanked her for knowing I needed an out. If I were to drive him there at all, I needed to imagine he was coming back home. I closed my eyes and remembered the smell of roses Dominic had always bought for me on this day—a rose for each year of our marriage.

I heard the sound of the boys' car in the driveway and hoped Dominic's angels would help me say the right things. I looked at my email, splattered with the day's heartache, and pressed send. The boys came into the house carrying boxes of pizza. It looked like we might be feeding half the street.

"How many pizzas did you get?"

"We'll finish them—easy!"

They started eating straight out of the box.

"Is Dad asleep?"

"Yes, he's tired. It's been a big day."

The conversation rolled out quite naturally. I told them what the palliative doctor had told me. Michael asked direct questions, including time frames. I told them everything. After lots of talking, Mike went to the computer and updated a select few of his closest friends.

Nicolas left the house. He went out to play poker with his friends and didn't say a word to any of them.

We attach hope to stories of recovery. We generally find it harder to bear stories about illnesses that are untidy, where nothing can be fixed, and the task is to love and let go. Not everyone is comfortable here. I had my own adaptations. To some, I was very open, but there were many times I had to deflect or package what I said, protecting myself from having to continuously pick up the emotional pieces of those around me who were falling apart, leaving bits of themselves everywhere.

A few days after talking with the boys, Patricia and I drove out to McCorely again to discuss Dominic's respite stay. Maggie welcomed us both and invited us into what looked like someone's private dining room. I half expected a platter of goodies to be brought in. The crocheted tablecloth reminded me of my grandmother; she had one that was almost identical. Her silver teapot and homemade ginger biscuits would have been perfect here. Maggie offered us something to drink, but as we talked, I felt the same shroud of cold descend that had enveloped me in the school office when I first disclosed our story.

Dominic's respite dates were confirmed. In three weeks, he would go in for a three-week stay. In the meantime, friends in Vancouver were fund-raising. Soon I would receive enough money to cover most of the costs of Dominic's nursing home care. The spirit of generosity and kindness showered on us from so many people in our life resides permanently in me.

Maggie's voice was calm. I tried to tune myself to it as she explained how respite worked. We would be welcome anytime and could stay the night if we wanted to. She said it would help if they had detailed knowledge of Dominic's daily routines, his likes and dislikes, so they could try to replicate them for him. They would like his care to be as age- and family-appropriate as possible and asked if they could arrange a home visit. They'd like to meet Dominic in his familiar environment and assess how they might best facilitate his adjustment.

We talked about the boys, and she agreed it would be a good idea for them to visit the nursing home with me before Dominic's stay. I hoped it might help alleviate some of the things they would struggle with when he was admitted—some of the imaginary thinking that can arise in all of us when we face the unfamiliar.

She explained how they might experience "body shock" at seeing such concentrated frailty in one place. In high-care nursing homes, this reality is not diluted by the rest of life. She explained how undergraduate nurses commonly experience body shock. A preliminary visit would be an opportunity to support the boys through this. Remembering Nic's reaction when Dominic was admitted to the psych hospital eight months ago, I was relieved to have this kind of help.

"Being in care is never the same as being at home," said Maggie.

I nodded.

Her face softened. "How do you think Dominic will manage without you?"

Such a thoughtful question; such a slap of reality sucking out my breath and rearranging my insides.

"I don't know.…This man is the love of my life. I'm not sure how we will live without each other."

Tears welled in her eyes.

A week later, the boys and I drove out to McCorely. Their last visit to an aged-care facility had been in Vancouver when they were about eight and nine years old. Their primary school visited residents in a nursing home once a month.

"Just go and chat to them," the teacher had said.

"About what?"

"Anything, but remember your manners."

These poor kids had no idea how to start, and whether the residents enjoyed them or simply tolerated them; the chance for meaningful interactions was never realized. The kids did not get the chance to see past wheelchairs and hairy chins or to learn to look with wonder into wrinkled faces filled with lines and lines of stories.

The boys knew I had been to visit several nursing homes for Dominic. They knew their dad needed increasing care. They knew this place was different from the nursing home they had visited as kids and that it was not a psych ward. I took Nic out of school. Michael did not have classes that day. He had cut down his uni courses to a bare minimum to help with Dominic's care at home, though I encouraged him to do one or two classes to keep connected to his friends.

"I don't know how much time we have left," he had said. "I want to be home more."

We approached the nursing home, one of several buildings sprawled out on thirty hectares of semirural surroundings. It was a newer building that contrasted with the old stone convent and the two beautifully maintained, heritage-listed Queenslanders dating back to the 1860s. We parked under a tree in front of a horse that was grazing noisily on the other side of a barbed wire fence. Glimpses of a new housing estate peeked through the trees.

Maggie was waiting for us. She introduced herself to Mike and Nic and led us back to the room with the table on which my grandmother's teapot could have sat. Emma, the recreational therapist who had patiently spent so much time with me on my very first visit to McCorely, joined us. An iPod wire dangled from Michael's left ear. I tugged at it, and he tucked the earphone in his pocket with a sideways look at me. The boys stood awkwardly in the room.

"Make yourselves comfortable, have a seat," said Maggie.

Chair legs groaned as they were dragged out from under the table.

I don't remember much of what was said that morning, but I remember how heavy the room felt. Michael did not say a word. Emma noticed, and Mike knew that Emma noticed. Like his dad, he was comfortable with silence, and today he was going to observe. Annoyed by questions inviting him out of his safe place of observation, he remained quiet and solemn. My boy was fundamentally sad.

Nic moved on his chair. He shifted his feet and, sitting up tall, he answered all the questions that were asked of him. They did this for each other, time and time again. I sat between them in that room holding sorrow and love together, watching as courage sat next to stillness.

"What would you like us to know about your dad that would help us to best look after him?"

"Dad really likes his music," said Nic.

"How will you cope with Queen blaring down the hallways?" I asked.

"Great choice—we'll probably join in! It'll be a refreshing change from 'The Fields of Athenry'!" said Maggie.

Laughter lightened the room. It gave us a doorway out.

"Would you like to see Dad's room?" I said to the boys.

Chair legs scraped against the floor. A resident passed us in the corridor. Her withered legs were folded at the knees, one in front of her and one to the side of her body, as she used her arms to slide her bottom forward along the floor. She didn't like being in a wheelchair but this way she could still get around. She moved comfortably along the floor with her legs folded up next to her in the shape of a Z. Nic moved toward me. I put my arm around him, and we walked on together. Maggie showed us to an empty room.

"Is this the exact room?" asked Nic.

"Yes," said Maggie.

"It's big."

"Like I said to your mum, we can bring beds in for you if you ever want to stay over. Feel free to bring in a beer or two and watch the footie"—rugby—"with your dad. Please tell me he supports the Wallabies?"

"Yeah, but never the English! You can't support the English in here!"

"Nor the All Blacks! This is serious Wallaby territory!" They had a small chuckle.

"Do you play rugby?" she said.

"Nah, got my head seriously smashed the one and only time I played."

"Do you play any other sport?"

"Soccer and basketball—except I've had concussions in soccer, so now Mom wants me to play chess!" He nudged me affectionately with his elbow. "We're all Manchester United fans. Dad's followed them since he was a kid. He told me he used to listen to the games on a little radio under the blankets in his bed when he was supposed to be asleep!" Michael smiled and walked quietly through the room, listening to the chatter as he stood in front of the bay window.

"The garden is really nice," he said. "It brings in lots of light."

"Would you like to walk through it?" said Maggie.

"Okay."

We walked on paths gently winding through manicured lawns past benches under shady trees and secluded patio spots where families or friends could visit together. Maggie showed us an undercover patio area with a barbecue. It looked out onto a natural forested area filled with gum trees.

"Feel free to have a barbie out here any time."

After strolling through the gardens, Maggie left us with Emma, who led us through more gardens to a recreational therapy cottage specifically set up for people with dementia. I had encouraged the boys to ask whatever was on their mind. Michael looked around, and his eyes grew sadder and deeper, sinking right into him. Nic did a visual scan: kitchenette for cooking, painting tables, crochet and knitting corner.

He didn't need long. He looked up from the arts and crafts table and met Emma's eyes.

"So, how *exactly* are you going to find something meaningful for my dad to do when he is surrounded by ninety-year-old women who like completely different things?"

We had reached the edge of what the boys could tolerate, and while the answer was reassuring, there was no pretending this would be easy.

"Can we just get outta here?" Michael mouthed to me.

It was time to leave. We drove from the nursing home to Mount Coot-tha's botanical gardens talking about everything but McCorely.

"Hey, can we go get the latest Madden game?" said Nic.

"Is it out yet?" I said.

"Yeah, you should see the graphics. They're awesome," said Mike.

"Sweet! I'm gonna kick Mitcho's arse!"

Nic and Mitch had a long history of playing Madden against each other. In Nic's words, they both rated themselves as "pretty much the best Madden players in Queensland," which meant serious competition between them. When one of them lost, the loser was irate.

I didn't have to watch the clock. My neuropsychologist Oktoberfest friend was at home with Dominic and would stay with him for as long as we needed her to.

"Don't rush home," she had said.

She and a few friends had given us a gift voucher for a meal at the restaurant in the gardens. Today was a perfect day to use it.

"I think they won me over," said Nic after ordering a steak.

"At McCorely?"

"Yeah. I liked that blonde chick."

"I liked that she didn't try to do a sell job on us," said Michael. "It's more honest. Makes it easier to trust the good stuff."

He appreciated their openness about this being a learning experience—that nursing Dominic, who was young, would be a new situation for the staff.

Michael and Nicolas were facing something most teenagers could not begin to imagine. No matter how perfect the place, their dad would still have to go to a nursing home. Nothing was going to make this bit better.

"Thanks for showing us the place," said Michael.

"Yeah, thanks. It sucks, but I think it's a good place," said Nic.

"I think they will be good to Dad there," said Mike.

Nic nodded.

I reached over the table and hugged them both.

"Are you crying?" said Nic.

"Mum cries at soppy commercials, of course she's crying!"

Genevieve came over the next evening for her night shift with Dominic and packed me off up the road to Bea's house to sleep. I came home the following morning at 5:45 a.m. I hadn't slept much, and there was no point in lying awake in someone else's bed. Genevieve was sitting out on the patio listening to the day wake up.

"Tea? Coffee?" I called from the kitchen.

"English Breakfast, please." She got up and joined me inside. "How did you sleep?"

"Not great."

"Honey, please tell me you're accepting a spot at McCorely?" She leaned against our kitchen counter waiting for the kettle to boil.

"Oh, it'll just be a temporary stay—you know, until exams are over."

She took both my hands in hers and looked me in the eyes. "Marie, as a friend who loves you, I'm going to put my nurse's hat on and tell you what could happen if you bring Dom home. He could have more laryngeal spasms. You've had to respond to a lot of them already. If one does not release by itself, he could choke and fall unconscious in front of the boys. You'll have to decide whether to call 000. If they arrive in time, the paramedics will have to do an assessment. With all the strange people, the equipment, the busyness, the noise, the ambulance—the entire sensory overload—Dominic will become scared and agitated and he won't be able to understand what is happening. They'll have to sedate him and take him to Emergency, even though everyone knows it's an environment he can no longer handle. You will not be able to stop this; they will take him there. His stress levels will skyrocket. It could induce more spasms. He could die a traumatic death. I know you don't want that for him. It could be your last memory of Dom, yours and the boys'. I know you don't want that for anyone."

She squeezed my hands.

"Marie, you have nursed Dom with all your love and dedication, with every ounce of your being. But you are exhausted, and he is too sick. It's dangerous for him to be at home now, he needs round-the-clock high-level nursing care, and you are not equipped here at home. McCorely will be good for all of you—it will be so much gentler than the possibility I have described. And, hopefully, it will give Dom a chance to die peacefully."

We had one more night at home together, and Nic came home from school that afternoon with some fantastic news. He had been named Dux of his school—the highest-ranking student in academic achievement. We were over the moon with excitement for him. Jack dropped by to congratulate him, and the three boys went off to play the new PlayStation game. Being Dux did not distract Nic from the latest Madden release; they had been riveted from the moment they'd bought it. Victory cries could be heard throughout the house, along with the sound of airborne bodies hurtling into each other, smashing helmets, frustrated protests, and spirited yells supporting Nic as his virtual character raced toward the end zone to score a touchdown.

It was still light outside, but the evening was just starting to greet the day. I lay on our bed next to Dom as he stared at the picture of the sun setting over the ocean that Max had hung on the wall the day little Lilly had written on the quilt. The picture was backlit and gave a realistic impression of water moving. It was not something we would normally have hung up in our home, but, as gaudy as it was, there was something hypnotic about it. The movement of the water mesmerized Dominic.

It also worked as a soothing night-light. Dominic did not like the dark anymore.

A little later, Jack popped his head into our bedroom.

"Hey!"

Dom raised his arm to say hello.

"Oi, something's missing!" Jack stepped into the room where he could get a better view. "You guys can't be watching a sunset like that without cocktails!"

He turned on his heels and disappeared. Fifteen minutes later he came back carrying five piña coladas on a silver tray.

"Oi, Mike! Nic!"

The boys came through to the bedroom.

"Now, this is how it's done!" he said and passed the tray around. Dominic grabbed the first glass and knocked it back without a splutter as the three boys climbed onto the bed and joined us for cocktails at sunset.

Jack looked worried. "I made an alcohol-free one for Dominic but he swigged down a different one—is that okay? Will it mess with his medication?"

"He's a man who knows how to celebrate!" I said. "That was thoughtful of you, but don't worry, he'll be okay!"

We raised our glasses.

"To Nic!"

"Hey, Dom, Nic's Dux!"

"FUCK NO!" said Dominic, disinhibited words of pride falling out of a smile so big they couldn't be contained.

"FUCK YES!" I said and raised my glass.

"FUCK YES!" said the three boys in unison.

Our glasses clinked, the house filled with celebratory laughter, and, for a time, we all forgot what was happening the next day.

I stroked the quilt and, before we knew it, it had wrapped itself around us. Cocktails, celebration, and quilt wrapping! What a sunset. What a last night at home.

The next morning Dominic leaned against the dresser in our bedroom. Calm and unpredictably lucid, he started talking about his illness.

He spoke of things he had done and about which he was embarrassed. He told me how scary it had been when he got lost overseas, how confusing it was not to understand the words people said, and how frustrating it was not to be able to speak properly. I heard the quieting of kitchen clatter as Nic listened in.

"I have dementia," Dominic said. "That's the problem."

He pulled me into his arms. *Oh no*, I thought—I was taking him to McCorely that morning. We had talked about it a few times before, but I never knew if he understood. When I asked him how he felt about going, he looked at me with eyes that told me he was still there.

"It's time," he said.

And then he was gone. He resumed pacing and asked if I could drive him to a store in a neighboring suburb to get a Vanilla Coke.

Nic came through, wide-eyed. "Random! What was that?"

I drove Dominic to the store, the complete opposite direction to the nursing home, and, with Vanilla Coke in hand, we finally made our way to McCorely. Maggie met us at the door. Dominic shook her hand with his melting fingers and smiled. She walked with us to his room, offering Dominic friendly chatter. He smiled at the softness in her voice and walked next to us with blank eyes, dragging his hand along the wall. The doctor would admit him a little later. In the meantime, Maggie gave us some time alone. Dominic lay on his bed and watched TV as I pottered about setting up his room. We had come armed with everything but the kitchen sink—anything that would make his room at McCorely feel more like home. Favorite photos, paintings I had done that he had always liked, our bed cover, music, a TV and DVD player, fresh flowers, the quilt, and a familiar stack of books he couldn't read anymore. We had always been surrounded by books at home, walls of them, just as I had been in my childhood home.

Later that afternoon, Sister Patricia drove out and found me balancing precariously on a chair while hanging up the quilt. It was too big for a single hospital bed, and Dominic wanted it on the wall. She grabbed the edge of the chair, stabilizing it for me, and begged me to climb down.

"Isn't it marvelous?" I leaned back with another chair wobble to have a look, and paid no attention to her increasing protests. It took up the whole wall. You couldn't get to Dom without being greeted by his story.

I felt like a quilt activist, but this quilt no longer needed me. It had long ago developed a life of its own. It demanded attention and invited us all into spaces we might otherwise have been too frightened to travel. The quilt had a voice. It spoke of Dominic's right to matter.

Patricia helped me unpack Dominic's clothes and then made herself at home in an armchair.

"You don't have to stay."

"You don't have to be alone when it's time to leave."

She paused.

"Besides which, I want to make sure you go home."

Genevieve and Felicity were waiting for me at home. I watched their mouths move without absorbing what they said. After they left, the boys and I ate a meal, a frozen one out of the freezer, probably pasta of some kind. We had an abundance of lasagna. We added a salad. We hung out and watched a bit of TV, or was it a DVD? We sat close together on the couch, bodies touching. Later, after everyone was in bed, Michael came through to my room.

"You look so small, Mum, so small in the bed all alone."

Six days later, one day short of a week, Maggie took me aside at McCorely. She was warm and friendly but soon got around to what she wanted to say. "What would you say if we offered Dominic a permanent bed?"

She saw my face freeze, and led me into the room I would always think of as a dining room.

"But...is he sick enough?"

She looked at me, treading gently. "He's sick enough."

"Really?"

She nodded.

"Have I just lost perspective?"

She did not agree or disagree.

"I don't know how you did this at home," she said.

The boys were not surprised, and were somewhat practical about the fact that Dom would not be coming home. They had been saying a slow and protracted goodbye to him over a long time. The sadness didn't change. They grieved deeply for their dad, but our home felt lighter now that the Green Goblin had moved out.

A couple of weeks later, as the reality sank in, Nic went on stage to receive his multiple awards at the school's prize-giving ceremony: a very courageous sixteen-year-old. The school hall exploded in applause when his name was read out. As he climbed the stairs onto the stage, he was greeted by a standing ovation.

I looked over at Mike, who was standing next to me with camera in hand. This time last year, he had gone through a very different graduation. Michael's Year 12 had unfolded against the backdrop of an undiagnosed and very scary time. Dominic had come to the graduation ceremony and, without all the support and understanding we had surrounding us here tonight, had caused him distress and public embarrassment. Unfazed by the memories of his ceremony, Mike was visibly proud of his brother.

If only you could see this, Dom. If only you could see them both in this moment.

As the sun set on this day of emotions mixed and stirred, Brother Neil caught my eye from the stage. He beamed us a smile before turning back to Nic with a hug and whispering something in his ear.

Prize-giving night was followed by an impressive school graduation dinner the next evening. The room sparkled with the exhilaration of boys launching into life after high school and the welling of parental tears saying goodbye to places we had once belonged. The sparkle of endings and new beginnings circled the room of white tables, floral centerpieces, moving speeches, a graduation DVD celebrating the school journey, and multiple toasts. The room went silent as the boys stood at their respective tables and raised their glasses to their families.

"To my mom *and* my dad," Nic said to the table. Then he turned to me. "Love ya, Mom. Thank you for *everything.*" The quiet was disrupted by a hall full of cheers. He held his look at me through the noise and smiled.

19

Graduation dinner ended late, and the next morning saw a mass exodus of thousands of Queensland school leavers making their way to the Gold Coast, their party central, just south of Brisbane. We drove to McCorely to see Dominic before heading down there. From wheelchairs and medication trolleys, the residents and nurses called out to wish Nic well.

"Don't let us see you drunk, like all those young mugs on TV!"

"You know the news cameras are out and about all the time!"

"Don't worry, we'll look after Mum. All mothers worry—it's their job."

"Off you go now, son. We know you won't be like the rest of them anyway!"

We said our goodbyes and I drove Nic to the Gold Coast. His friends were already there. Five of them were sharing an apartment. Before I left them to experience this strange rite of passage together, I checked out the apartment, reminded Nic to make his daily phone calls home, checked out their plan for looking out for each other, told them all to call if there were any problems day or night, and watched their eyes slowly glaze over as I obsessed about covering all the bases.

"Serious? Call you every day?"

"Yup, very serious. We've been through this, Nic."

"I'll defs text."

"Texts are great in addition to the call, and if I don't hear your actual voice by the set time, I'm driving down, so you have to decide which option is worse."

I gave Nic a hug and a kiss.

"Bye, Marie," said Mitch.

"Bye, Mitcho." He got a hug and a kiss from me, too.

"We're cool," he said. "We'll look out for each other. You and Mum talked, I know, 'cause you both said exactly the same things."

I left their apartment smiling and grabbed myself a takeout coffee. I walked to the car and threw out a prayer of protection for my boy during this wild week of partying. Pictures of drunken school leavers in fistfights and vomiting in gutters on national TV didn't help. I made my way back home along the busy highway. I had an hour to myself in the car. I cranked up the latest *So Frenchy So Chic* CD and sipped away at my coffee, skipping over a couple of tracks to play the ones I liked. As I neared home, I stopped at the supermarket to pick up some dog food. We were out of milk, too. The music cut out mid-song as I parked the car and switched off the ignition.

I trawled the aisles without a list and popped things into the cart, pondering what to make for dinner. It would only be Mike and me. I saw the shelves of bottled water and wondered if Nic would drink as much water as he would alcohol over the next week. I strolled past washing detergents, household cleaners, and magazines splashing out trashy headlines, and made my way to the pet food aisle. I stood there looking for the usual brand of kibble. They had been moved—no doubt a marketing ploy to force shoppers to notice other products. I scanned the shelves for the familiar red-and-black packaging and felt a tap on my shoulder. I turned to see someone I didn't know very well greeting me with a somewhat overzealous "Hi!" I had met her once or twice through a previous workplace. She called her husband over and introduced him to me.

"This is Marie. Remember, I told you about Dominic? She's his wife," she said.

"Oh! Yes. I'm sorry," he said, shaking my hand. At first I thought his little frown might be one of concern.

"So, your husband doesn't know who he is anymore?" He leaned forward as if to get closer to the intrigue. "And he does strange things? He's not really normal anymore, is he?"

I'm not sure that assumptions punctuated with question marks qualify as questions. It felt more like he was hoping to get a peek into a freak show through a conversation filled with juicy details.

"I guess it depends on how you look at things," I said, maintaining eye contact. "Besides which, what is normal anyway?"

I was calm and did not disguise the challenge, but I was too tired to take them on, and they seemed to have less insight than most green goblins, so what was the point? They looked at me, waiting for the gossip.

I took a deep breath, giving life to what I knew of love and normality. I politely moved on despite wanting to lecture, rant, and rave at them until they disappeared yelping under the heavy bags of dog food.

What *is* normal anyway? A construct, I know, but I went home and looked up the origin of the word. I searched through dictionaries, good old Google, *Webster's Word Histories*, disability texts, and, some time later, *The Disability Studies Reader*, edited by Lennard Davis, and the work of Jane Hutton, a colleague who has written about ideas of normality. From what I could find, the word "normal" derived from the Latin *norma* and originally meant "perpendicular." It referred to the forming of a right angle, the angle made according to a carpenter's square. It was, at its root, a mathematical term. The square provided a way for a carpenter to regularly reproduce the same angles and corners. Over time, the use of the word "normal" evolved, and it was used in a more generalized, less literal sense to mean "according to rule." It was from this understanding that most meanings of the current word "normal" are derived, but when, in the mid-1800s, the word was defined and generally understood to mean "conforming to common standards; usual, even natural," we began to use it as a way to evaluate people and their actions rather than angles.

I guess if "normal" now describes what is "usual, even natural," we might not notice the rich range of storylines that contribute to the life of a person we are measuring. We wouldn't even look for them, as we would have constructed an unquestionable absolute that comes hand in hand with a set of ready-made expectations.

I drove back to see Dominic that afternoon, still ranting away at the couple at the supermarket in my head. In my imagination, they remained trapped under bags of dog food, wishing they had never greeted me in the first place. I was waving a carpenter square at them, reminding them that linking ill health and notions of human worth is not a new discriminatory assumption. Could they not see that they were subscribing to socially constructed ideas of normality that tend to accept, even revere, those who fit the square and marginalize those of us who do not measure up? And as for ideas of abnormality, the problem was less about "not really being normal anymore" and more about how the construction of normalcy itself has created difficulties for people with disabilities. What about the richness of life they were missing out on by upholding these generalized notions of what it means to be normal—a normal man or woman, a normal family, a normal husband, a success, a failure, a normal sick person, and a sick person who is not normal? Ugh!

It was true that the Dominic we knew had changed. I noticed people watching him as if he were already a memory and wondered what that was like for him. He no longer met expectations according to the "common standards" and he had lost many of the abilities our culture values as important. But did this mean he no longer had a sense of self? Does that ever really go away?

If identity is coconstructed in acts of living with others, then, "normal" or not, I don't believe a sense of self disappears. The African philosophy of *ubuntu* describes this beautifully. Translated, *ubuntu* means "I am because we are." It holds that we are interconnected in each other's humanity, that our sense of self is shaped within our relationships—by the people with whom we share life. It suggests a sense of unity between people through which we discover more about ourselves.

I pulled up at McCorely, an article on the politics of disability penned in my head, and parked the car in my usual spot. I watched the same friendly horse grazing on the other side of the fence. He swished his tail casually. I left my imaginary conversation and the carpenter square in the car and walked through the various corridors to get to Dominic's room. He was standing at the side of his bed.

"Hi," I said softly so as not to startle him. He stiffly opened both arms. I walked into them and they closed around me. He didn't speak. Then he dropped his arms and walked over to the quilt hanging on the wall. He stood there quietly. He ran his hand over the picture of the boys smiling through face paint he had painted on them with a message for me on Mother's Day. He stroked their colorful faces and laid both palms over them. I watched him hold them.

Dominic moved his hands across the fabric to the picture of me in my wedding dress, the same block he had reacted to with Felicity. He gently traced his finger over the outline of my face. He lingered there and then turned to me. I took his hand. Dominic could not find his words that day but, once again, we had found each other. His face crumpled as he cried without tears. Then the moment was gone. The pacing resumed, but I was left in no doubt as to what gave Dominic life. He paced the corridors of McCorely with the three of us still firmly imprinted on the palms of his hands.

20

"Hello, love," said Sister Philomena. She was ensconced in a comfy chair in a sunny spot in the nursing home lobby. Residents were used to seeing me every day and often greeted me with smiles or a touch and endearing chitchat of some kind. "Do I look okay?"

She supported herself on the arms of the chair, stood up slowly, and turned around so I could see her from every angle. Her hair was newly set and the light shining through the window highlighted a subtle tint of purple I had not noticed the day before. She stroked the shoulder of her bolero jacket. It matched, perfectly, the midnight blue in her creaseless dress. I wondered why she had asked for my opinion. I was hardly an icon of style in my faded shorts and T-shirt.

"It's new, you know."

"What's the occasion?"

"One of us has gone to God. I'm going to the funeral this morning. We're just waiting for a lift to the chapel and I want to look my best."

"Oh, I'm sorry…"

"She was ready, love, and she was very sick. What do you think of my dress?"

"The color is beautiful on you; the blue brings light to your eyes."

"Thanks!"

She used both arms to support herself as she lowered herself back into the chair. The residents who were able to attend the funeral congregated together, waiting for their ride to the chapel next to the old convent on the grounds. Funerals were a part of life at McCorely. Saying goodbye was familiar. Death was certain. Life was running its course, and everyone would eventually leave here this way. I wondered how much residents reflected on this time of their lives—those of them who could. Death is certain for all of us. Most of us don't think about it much, but in this place, life was completing its circle.

Sister Philomena was Dominic's neighbor from across the hall. She had been a brilliant musician. "Violin mostly," she had told me when she had first invited me into her room and showed me around. "But I taught piano as well."

She couldn't stand anything out of tune; it upset her ears, she said.

"It's unfair, you know; he is so young," she chatted on, changing the subject. "Me...it makes sense that I am here, but..." She shook her head. "Do you ever ask why?"

I shrugged. I have tried to release questions like this into the sky, to hang out in space with all the other questions of the world that have no answers.

"Sometimes there are no explanations," I said.

Sister Philomena was a Sister of Mercy who had taken a vow of poverty but, given the chance, I think she would have shopped until she dropped. I'm not sure how she managed back in the days of the habit.

I often wonder if she snuck on something silky or luxurious under her robes. Her hair was always perfect, even after a snooze. She showed me the trick, a not so subtle hint that I could do better than my usual, more windswept and casual look. She slept on a pink satin pillowcase.

"Feel it," she said as she caressed her hand over it. "It prevents that dry bed-hair tangle at the back of your head."

I stroked her pillow.

"And it's best to have two so that when one is in the wash, you always have another."

She had a soft spot for us, despite her more aloof reputation. I had an invitation to pop in and visit her in her room anytime, a privilege not offered to many, she said. She had an iron and an ironing board. She would let me use it if I wanted, but I was under strict instructions not to tell anyone. She didn't want everyone and their dog coming to ask if they could use her iron. Hers was a really good quality one.

She popped in to see Dominic every now and then. She didn't stay—she would simply knock on his door and bring us homemade muffins.

A friend made them for her, and without fail, she'd keep four aside for us.

Being neighbors, we would see each other quite a bit. Our conversations were mostly about music, a particular resident who annoyed her more than anything when she sang out of tune, new clothes and whether they matched, or the next shopping expedition she hoped to enjoy. So, despite my everyday casual appearance, I guess I wasn't too surprised by her request for approval in the lobby. After admiring her new dress, I said goodbye and made my way up to Dominic's room.

Robbie Williams's voice sang out down the corridor, drowning out the familiar squeaks of wheelchairs. Queen and Josh Groban had taken a temporary backseat to Robbie, who was in Brisbane for two concerts. His music was being churned out on every radio station, so, thanks to Dominic and a nurse who had given him a *Robbie in Concert* DVD, the elderly residents living in Dominic's wing had no choice but to swap their Irish lilts for a bit of pop. I'm sure Sister Philomena was pleased by the break from Queen. While both Robbie and Freddie can hold a good tune, I imagine our musical nun much preferred the lyrics of "Angels" to those of "Fat Bottomed Girls."

The boys joined us at McCorely a couple of hours later, by which time "Angels" was on its fifteenth replay.

"Hey, guys, guess what?" said Nic.

"What?"

"We got tickets to the Robbie Williams concert next week!"

"How did you manage that!?"

Nic explained that one of his teachers had called. A charity foundation had given the school tickets to the concert, including backstage passes. They were offered to Mike and Nic. Mike immediately gave his ticket to me.

"No way, you guys go. It'll be fun."

"C'mon, Mum, you love Robbie Williams, you should go." There was no way I would take his ticket, and anyway, I didn't want to leave Dominic's side.

"This is ridiculous! You need to have some fun, too. That's what you say to us. You should go. C'mon."

They stepped out into the corridor but I could still hear them talking.

"You call them."

"No, you call them."

"But you're much better at this sort of thing."

"Fine. You got the number?"

Within five minutes, they had arranged extra tickets. Nic had told the charity foundation organizers that I needed a break and asked if there was another ticket available.

"Sweet as! You're going!" said Mike as they came back into the room.

"Yeah," said Nic, putting his phone back in his pocket. "Our show is full but we got you two tickets to the show the night after ours."

A week later, the boys made their way to the concert and watched Robbie Williams rock the stadium.

On the other side of Brisbane, I lay on the nursing home bed with Dominic, waiting for him to drift off to sleep before I headed home. My phone started to vibrate on the bedside table. I managed to reach over Dominic without disturbing him too much and answer it. A thunderous noise came down the line, with two voices trying to shout over it.

"Hey, Mom, listen!"

"Mum, can you hear us? This one's for Dad."

The boys were standing in the crowd with phone held up high. I put my phone on speaker for Dominic to hear.

"He's singing it for you," I whispered. Dominic smiled, not because of the boys' gesture—that smile came from me—but because the music reached him, and to Dominic, Robbie and the fifty-two thousand, four hundred and thirteen members of the crowd were singing "Angels" especially for him.

Dom had never had any musical training. He never played an instrument or sang in a choir. But music seemed to enchant him, and it opened up another doorway for all of us once he fell into the clutches of the Green Goblin. When Dom had been at home with us, we put all of Queen's songs onto the boys' computers. That way, when Dominic paced into their rooms with repetitive and annoying questions, they could redirect his attention to Freddie Mercury and sing together. Dominic's incessant pacing and tedious questions required the patience of Job. Daniel once described it as "Chinese torture." He worried it would wear down our nerves and wondered how we managed. Sometimes we didn't. But the music helped.

Like the day when Dominic bopped stiffly, on his pacing route, to "We Will Rock You." Michael turned up the volume so that Dom could hear it wherever his pacing took him. Freddie's voice belted out of his room. As the next track came on, Dominic returned to Michael's room and asked him to play the track again. He asked for it to be played over and over, he merged with the rhythm, and from his frozen face, where muscles no longer responded, his usually empty eyes sparkled with light. Freddie got us on a good day. The four of us spontaneously started singing, stamping our feet, and clapping. *Stamp, stamp, clap. Stamp, stamp, clap. Stamp, stamp, clap. Stamp, stamp, clap.*

We were having fun, the kind of spontaneous fun that we remembered from our *lives* before dementia. The chorus got extra volume out of us.

STAMP, STAMP, CLAP. STAMP, STAMP, CLAP.

After about the tenth replay, Michael's mobile rang.

"Hey, mate!" Jack yelled into the phone. "Turn the bloody music down—what are you doing playing the same song over and over? It's driving me nuts!"

Mike laughed and cranked the music up louder.

"Dude! We're having a rock concert with Dad."

"Oh. Cool!"

The song rang through our heads for days. I even heard Felicity humming it as we worked on the quilt. Jack had filled them in, she said, and they had joined in that day, rocking with us from their house. *Stamp, stamp, clap. Stamp, stamp, clap.*

Other than the song "Angels," Robbie became a passing phase. Queen and Josh Groban remained firm favorites, although Dominic didn't seem to need the volume as loud anymore. While time in the nursing home rolled over for him with no sequence or carryover from one moment to the next, there was something about music that gave us another way to be together. I will always carry close to my heart the image of Michael singing to Dominic at McCorely. Michael has a beautiful singing voice but doesn't show it off; very few people have heard it. I watched him many times, sitting on Dominic's bed, singing gently as the music in his voice called out to his dad. Dominic joined in with no inhibitions. Fixing his gaze on his son, he would follow Michael's words as they moved their hands in time, conducting an invisible orchestra in tune with the beat of their hearts.

Music enlarged Dominic's existence. The more he lost the abilities of abstraction and language, the more his sensory response to music seemed to grow. He would close his eyes and inhale the sounds, responding to music in ways that left me convinced I had seen the shiver in his soul.

Certain music evoked in Dominic a surge of emotion so powerful it left him weeping. Josh Groban stirred up an almost primal response. It was tender, raw, and full. There was something magical in Josh's voice that enabled Dominic to express himself. He showed emotions, he felt deeply, and he could find and understand words. Not only that, he could memorize the words and melodies of whole new songs, singing them as if he'd known them forever.

One evening, I put on Josh Groban's CD *Awake*. It was a newly released album, and despite having only heard the songs once or twice before, Dominic was already singing the words fluently. He sat in a chair in the bay window in his room. Dusk was turning the sky purple and the clouds milky gray. The trees lost their daylight shadows, slowly transforming into silhouettes. We were alone. As the music played, Dominic started to sing.

His melting throat muscles threw out a flat sound, but the words fluttered gently into my lap. He sat stiffly on the edge of his chair and reached for my hand. He sang the song word for word as if it were his own heart's song. He stopped once, right near the beginning. "I'm singing this to you," he said. He held my look, his eyes not leaving mine, until the whole song was sung.

She stares through my shadow
She sees something more
Believes there's a light in me
She is sure
And her truth makes me stronger
Does she realize
I awake every morning

With her strength by my side
I am not a hero
I am not an angel
I am just a man
Man who's trying to love her
Unlike any other
In her eyes I am

21

Each day, when I drove out to see Dominic at McCorely, I hung my coat of grief on a tree branch outside the front door. Doing so helped him to breathe. Dom remained so finely tuned to the emotions of others that any stress, no matter how cleverly hidden, would leap out and stick to his body like small iron filings to a magnet. So, calm and gentle, we enjoyed the richness of being and the gift of doing nothing, while grief waited quietly in the trees. When he fell asleep at night, I went outside, picked up the old, familiar coat, and sobbed all the way home.

McCorely had a rhythm of its own. Weekdays were busier. Visitors, volunteers, and families walked in and out of the automatic glass doors of the front entrance. Nurses came and went as their shifts began and ended. Dominic's favorite nurse cycled in. She was from China, studying in Australia for her master's degree. Sometimes I'd see them from the main foyer, walking together through the recreation area, past the chapel, inside and outside, around and around. "We're walking the Great Wall of China," she would say, and Dominic would laugh. Different days would see groups gathered in the foyer ready to go out somewhere—the beach, the wetlands, shopping maybe. I heard the friendly chatter as they were helped into the bus and pushed in wheelchairs, or independently refused a hand even when one was not offered. Doctors visited on Wednesdays.

They went from room to room, nurses by their side with trolleys and charts. Dominic would leave the room whenever they entered. Up and out he walked, straight past them, without so much as a look. He would have nothing to do with doctors. He would see no one accept Dr. Liam, but Dr. Liam was too far away now and couldn't visit.

It was different with Maggie. He would glide into her office, near the front entrance, several times a day. He never lost his way there. Her door was always open and her desk perpetually crowded with piles of paperwork. Dom had a ghostlike way of appearing and greeting her with a wide grin, staring at her expectantly, completely unaware of whether or not he had interrupted her. As the director of care, she ran a busy show, but I would often find him there looking at framed photos of her family, or sitting with her in front of the computer as she read him emails Daniel had sent to him. I asked her once if it bothered her.

"Not at all," she said in her usual unruffled way. "Dominic is a young man who until recently worked and had his own office. My office is an environment he knows."

Almost every day I would see people gather around the kitchenette in Dominic's cluster, making tea and eating various goodies baked in the kitchens that day: muffins, brownies, sweet slices of different kinds.

I frequently found Sister Agnes, Sister Mary Catherine, Nelly, and Sister Eunice there, chatting and helping others less able.

One morning, as I walked past this group of women, Sister Agnes sang out, "We're all looking out for your Dominic."

"Thank you, Sister."

"We saw the boys go by. Would you like a cuppa? I'll bring it up to you in Dominic's room."

She poured me a cup before I had the chance to answer and so I stopped by to chat. Having a young family here was new for them, but Dominic was also only the third man ever to have entered McCorely.

"You know, when the first man entered here," she said with a cheeky smile, "he said to me, 'Sister, I'm the only man here.' You know what I said to him? 'And blessed art thou among women!'"

Guffaws of laughter and thunderous applause filled the kitchenette.

It was a kind and a very different world, one where we belonged but didn't really fit. I finished my tea and friendly chat and made my way up to Dom's room.

"Olive grabbed me this morning and wouldn't let go," said Mike as I walked in. "It's kind of freaky."

"She tugs on our shirts and walks with us, crying loudly right up in our face. What are we supposed to do?" said Nic.

Olive lived at McCorely. She had dementia, too. In her younger days, she and her husband had been foster parents to several children. She was a religious Catholic woman who felt most connected to her sense of self when she was caring for others.

"Danny won't let me take care of him," she would complain to me.

She called Dominic by a number of names: Danny, Devon, Daryl, Dillon. She was frustrated that she couldn't look after him, and every time this happened, she told me she wanted to catch the bus home to her husband. She started to cry and asked me for fifty cents for the bus.

We came up with a plan to get past Olive.

The main entrance was not locked during the day. I was told Dominic often looked for me when I wasn't there and waited at the front door of the building for me to arrive. He had been fitted with a bracelet that would activate a sensor for staff, alerting them every time he walked out the front door. He didn't usually wander far—mostly he headed out to the driveway to see if I was there—but waiting was hard for him. He walked in and out, in and out, setting off the sensor copious times, waiting on the move. On one of these days, Olive was there, too, waiting for the bus.

She got to me before Dominic, and tugged on my sleeve. Dom took one look at this and bolted back to his room.

I slowed down and walked with her so that the boys could leave me and catch up with Dominic.

"I've got a rosary," she said, clutching my arm. I stopped walking, saw Dom and the boys disappear around the corner, and had a closer look at the rosary beads she was holding. They were warm and sweaty from the grip of her palm.

"Olive, do you think if you said the rosary for Dominic it would help him?"

"Oh yes! But not in my room. I'm not staying here! After the rosary, I'm going home."

She took me by the hand and led me, with determination, to her room. She dragged a chair out into the corridor.

"I'm not staying in my room!"

The old familiar beads hung from her fingers as she sat on her chair out in the corridor and started to softly pray for Dom.

"Thanks, Olive."

She nodded, without interrupting the whisper of her Hail Mary.

I left her praying in the corridor and made my way toward Dominic's room.

Before I got there, Mike and Nic came strolling down the corridor toward me, clad in their low-riding, undie-showing shorts. Led by Dominic's urgent desire to pace, they were already walking up and down, supporting him with a walking belt clipped around his hips. The physiotherapist had shown us all how to use this wide padded belt with handholds to assist Dom from sitting to standing, and to stabilize and support him while walking. They wandered through the corridors, out toward the gardens, with Dom in his harness, one on either side of him. Sporting fashionably chaotic hair and laughing with Dom when he said "the lamest" things, they were quite unaware of how touching their being with him was to onlookers as life shifted into a sadder, fuller kind of waiting time.

Later that night, back at home, I stepped over an array of clothes that covered Michael's bedroom floor. Beth was with Dominic. She came once a week for an afternoon-to-bedtime "shift" so that I could be at home and attend to the rest of life. Michael's newly washed T-shirts, jeans, and gym clothes lay intertwined with all the dirty ones. It was just a matter of time before he put the whole lot through the washing machine again, rather than sift through what needed to be put away and what should be washed.

"Hey," I said.

"Hey."

I handed him a cup of tea and sat on the crumpled duvet at the end of his bed. He threw me a pillow to tuck behind my back as I leaned against the wall. He wrapped his fingers around his mug of tea, threw his long legs over mine, and looked up to the ceiling where his thoughts were taking shape.

"You know, I feel like Dad is making the ultimate sacrifice for me," he said.

"What do you mean?"

"This is changing me..."

I sipped my tea and waited.

"It's like I'm learning stuff, stuff I wouldn't be thinking about if this weren't happening....Dunno what it is yet, but I want something good to come out of it, you know? For Dad's sake, so it's not all for nothing."

I stroked his bare foot.

"Aah! Your hand's freezing!"

I warmed my hands on my cup of tea and went back to holding his foot.

"It's weird," he said. "People say things like this make you stronger, but it's..."

"I don't know if this will make me stronger," Nic interrupted from his bedroom, "but I *do* know it will make me different."

He was lying on his bed, propped up on one elbow, reading the latest *Manchester United* magazine. They lay on their beds, where they could see each other, sharing wisdom spared from clichés.

God doesn't give you anything you can't cope with. What won't kill you will only make you stronger.

These bare offerings were essentially unhelpful. Nietzsche said the latter and he died of madness! This illness was hideous.

"The worst of the worst diagnoses anyone could ever get," said Nic.

Offering us clichés like get-better pills was no help to us at all—they were a dose of empty platitudes.

The next morning, back at McCorely, we saw Dominic, wearing his T-shirt from Stradbroke Island, laughing with the nurses about the slogan scrawled across his chest: "No crocs here, sharks ate 'em all." He said it over and over again, inviting the laughter to continue. The boys watched their dad express the delight of a child. Dominic's laughter was joyous. There was comfort in knowing he was happy, but that day, it was a reminder of what this illness was doing. The laughter—the jokes and the silly slogan—made their dad feel good, but it was not funny or touching for them. They had to step away.

Leaving to go home was a delicate act. Sometimes we had to sneak out.

If Dominic didn't see us leave, he experienced no distress, so we learned a game of kind and affectionate distraction. But it was uncomfortable, like putting clothes on that didn't fit, clothes that were too small and constantly chafed at your body.

"I hate this. It feels like a trick. I have to deceive my own dad," said Nic.

"Love you, Dad," the boys would say to Dominic, kissing him. He liked the sound of his name; the reassurance released a smile of recognition from his stiffening face. They would wait a few minutes and then slip out of the room. No one said, "Bye, Dad, we're going home now."

I stayed with him. On their way out, the boys would call a nurse to let her know I needed help. A nurse would pop in and distract Dominic, usually with the offer of a walk. Most times he agreed and joined her, walking past me without a flinch and not noticing when I slipped out once he had left his room. But sometimes he outwitted us by getting to the front door before we did, insisting he join us.

"Oh, I left something in your room. Do you mind if we go back to get it?" I would say. He would nod and, hand in hand, we would stroll back, hang out for a bit, and then try the whole thing all over again while the boys waited in the car. This was as much a strategy to soothe the boys as it was for Dominic. Leaving a distressed dad who wanted to come home at the door did not make for a good night's sleep.

We started parking at the back of the building and leaving through a staff door Dom did not know about. We had more success when the boys came in a separate car. They didn't have to wait for me to go home, and it made for easier goodbyes.

One weekend, the boys were out with friends and I was alone with Dominic when the doctor was called in to see him. The doctor had been gardening at home when he got the call. He drove straight in, still wearing his gardening boots. I really liked that. There was something earthy about it, something grounded and real, familiar yet unusual in a setting like this—but then, so were we.

Dominic's lungs were filling with fluid and muck, and his muscles were not strong enough to cough everything up. ALS was choking the life out of him, and dementia drove him to pace in a body that was melting. Providing what medical relief there was for one of these illnesses usually caused problems for the other. These two diseases, while linked, were in constant battle with each other.

I wrote to my family.

Sometimes, in the middle of this tangle, there are pauses filled with moments that are deeply touching, a sort of intense undiluted time where we pack it all in before it is lost again. Here, love and sadness seem so intertwined. I can't help thinking that while we are losing Dominic, we are also seeing more of him.

Today, we spoke of not fighting this and letting go. About how I loved him; how much we would miss him. That as the boys grew older, they would always know him. That I'd be there for them; all of you and our friends would, too. That we would look out for each other—we would all be okay. He seemed to need to know this.

I lay holding his frail body in my arms until he fell asleep, and I wondered if the ability to remember is less important than the knowledge that you will be remembered. Then I whispered to him. I asked, once he was gone, if he could find a way to let me know he was okay.

"Dad's not eating much anymore," said Michael one evening.

"You know how we're not going to do PEG feeds or put Dad on a machine?" said Nic.

I nodded.

"Will he starve to death?"

"No, sweetheart…"

"That would be terrible," he said before I could continue.

"Dad won't starve; he won't even feel hungry."

Mike listened in.

"How do we know for sure?"

"I was worried about it, too, so I asked about it. The doctor told me that when people are dying, they gradually lose the urge to eat and drink, and this releases endorphins, which helps them to feel more comfortable. It's the body's way of making it easier."

"So Dad won't feel it? He won't get hungry at all?"

"He won't feel hungry or thirsty, and not eating will cause him no pain. Forcing him to eat food could make him feel sicker. As the body shuts down people sometimes just slip into a coma and die quite peacefully."

It was not how we were used to doing things. Food is a way to nurture and show we care. When people are sick, we make chicken soup and encourage them to eat. Our way of caring had shifted to letting Dominic eat when he wanted to and to accepting that sometimes he didn't want to eat a thing.

"Would you like to talk to the doctor about it? He might have more answers for you than I have."

"It's cool. You're good at explaining this stuff. I just....I don't want dad to suffer."

A few days later, Mike and Nic climbed into Ed's pickup and the three of them drove off to the dump. Ed had spent time with the boys at home, helping with household maintenance and a general cleanup. Along with our garden refuse and household junk, the pickup was crammed with accumulated frustration and the tension of long-term sorrow. Ed felt the weight of their suffering. They arrived at the dump with dust blowing; it was a windy day. Nic leaned against the open door; Mike didn't want to get out of the car.

Ed said nothing.

He picked up a brick from among the refuse and held it for a few seconds, weighing it in his hand, then smashed it through an old TV. The boys' eyes widened. Ed found an old toaster, a four-slice version, and hurled it across the dump. It bounced off bits of discarded life before the metal housing shattered into several mangled pieces.

Michael stepped out of the car.

Ed picked up a broken stool and flung it at an old mattress that lay convex, springs protruding through its pierced chest. Michael walked slowly toward a stack of small concrete blocks. He picked one up and hurled it at a nearby computer, smashing the screen to smithereens. Before long, the three of them were at it. Raging, destroying, running, laughing, and whooping, they emptied the pickup bed and demolished old appliances and other household goods until the energy expelled itself. The pickup was considerably lighter on the ride home.

It was time for another respite break. I packed the car with beach gear—items that would nurture vulnerable spirits—and took the boys to Straddie with Jack and Mitch. Beth gave me a copy of Leunig's *The Curly Pyjama Letters,* a fictional collection of whimsical letters written between two friends, Vasco Pyjama and Mr. Curly, who lived near Curly Flat. The shape of life was changing. In moving from the madness of Wonderland into the more reflective world of Curly Flat, I adopted a quirky phrase of Vasco's: in all the variations of wobbly life, Beth became my own "gargling angel," looking out for me. She spent time with Dominic during the respite week, and phoned daily to reassure me that he was okay, saying whatever it took to encourage me to stay the full week away rather than just a few days. Everything at McCorely was fine. Dominic was fine. He could feel angels around him, he told her. It was me she was worried about.

I wrote to my family when we got back from the island.

You know, in some way, the boys are a great balancer. These respite breaks are so important for them and, if I'm honest, I don't think I would take time away just for myself. The Green Goblin would consume all of me.

Images of Dominic struggling to breathe started to enter my dreams.

I woke in the night gasping, trying to breathe for him. Mornings were better. Whatever darkness the night had delivered dissolved in the brightness that love brought in the next day.

Despite his deterioration, when Dominic saw me today, he stopped his pacing, smiled right back to his ears, and said, "Hello, my beautiful!"

We also had Queen. Long dead, Freddie Mercury still worked his magic, accompanying Mike and Nic as they competed against each other in daily push-up competitions on the floor in Dominic's room. Dominic gave them a thumbs-up from the bed. This room looked more like a musical boot camp than death's waiting room.

One morning, Mitch came to visit and joined in. Nic was determined to outdo Mitch's push-up score. He closed his eyes in an attempt to ignore Mitch's jibes and distractions. No way would he fall prey to the disruptive ploys. As he reached an equal score, Nic finally gave in to laughter.

"You bastard!" he said, collapsing on the linoleum floor.

Dominic started to laugh.

Mike changed the music to Josh Groban.

"Look!" Michael nudged Nic with his foot.

Dominic had climbed out of bed, put his arms around me, and started to dance.

I closed my eyes and stepped into the feel of him—the way he used to tread on my toes when we danced; the way we would spoon at night, even after a fight; the way he played with my hair. In the simple, synchronous movement of our bodies, Dominic exuded the gentleness of spirit I had always known and, once again, he held me as though I was sacred.

I did not see a head pop into the doorway and discreetly step away.

Dominic's room now housed four beds. One bed was set up permanently next to his. When it didn't get in the way, we could push them together like a double bed. We decided on mattresses for the boys. That way we could move them easily if they were not needed. They were set up, out of Dominic's way, on the floor in the alcove of a bay window that looked out into the garden. A photo of the four of us wrapped up in the quilt, taken on that memorable piña colada evening, hung on the wall in a bright orange frame with a pendant dangling over it. My dad had spent hours making this gorgeous pendant from delicate flowers he had pressed and set in clear resin. It was beautifully arranged, with a specific flower representing each one of us.

When I had read my dad's letter to Dominic, I did not know if he understood it. But, lying on the bed together and holding the pendant, Dominic pointed to the flowers one by one.

"Me…you…Mike…Nic."

He had pointed to the framed family photo, asking me to hang it there.

"Cool pendant," said Michael when he arrived alone the following morning. He took the pendant off the photo and lay sprawled across the bed with Dominic, holding it in his hand.

"Me…Mum…you…Nic," said Dominic, pointing to it.

Michael smiled through his hangover. He had had a big night. Maggie couldn't interest him in greasy bacon and eggs. He settled for toast. Aged care is never the same as home. That said, what other place would offer a hungover teenager recovery food as he lay in bed with his dying dad?

"I've got a present for you," Michael said to Dominic.

He opened the covers of the book *Dear Dad: Father, Friend, and Hero,* a tribute to dads filled with photographic images of animals reflecting love and humor. Dominic listened to the tender melody in Michael's voice. Michael moved closer to Dominic, showed him the poem he had written inside the front cover, and, sharing the same pillow, read it to him.

I arrived with Nic a few hours later and found Michael and Dominic snoozing lightly together. I had been giving Nic another driving lesson. We were past the stage of driving around empty parking lots and had hit the streets, starting on the quiet residential streets of Samford, a semirural community with houses on acreages and hardly any traffic—except for one day when there was a dad out there with his teenage daughter, doing exactly the same thing.

"Whoa! She's hot!"

"Keep your eyes on the road."

"See that? She was checking me out."

"Nic, left side of the road. You're swerving; keep to the left."

He laughed and steered the car back to the left. "Yeah, well, she's swerving, too!"

"Hey, slow down. You'll fail the test outright if you speed."

We drove up the hill to where the road flattened out into a narrow cul-de-sac, got through a six-point turn, and whizzed back down the hill, building up speed toward the stop sign while the blonde stalled her hill start on the other side of the road.

"Slow down, slow down, slow down, there's a stop sign," I said, pushing down on an imaginary brake pedal.

"Mom!"

"Stop, stop, stooopppp!"

"What?!" He screeched to a halt and we both fell forward into the restraint of our seat belts. "Geez, Mom! You scared me!"

Soon, we upgraded to busy streets with double lanes, winding turns, yield signs, busy roundabouts, train crossings, ongoing yelps at stop signs, and, finally, driving out to McCorely.

Michael heard us enter. He lifted his woolly head, propped himself up on his elbow, and asked how the drive went.

"No stalls, and I nailed the hill starts."

"Cool."

"I wanna show Dad—what do you think?"

"Hey, where did he go?"

"Probably walking again." Nic went to find him. "Hey, Dad, wanna go for a drive?"

Dominic followed us out to the car. Nic put his learner plates back up on the front and back windscreens while Michael and I helped Dominic into the car. Michael sat with him in the backseat. Nic started the engine, a purr of a start, and drove very slowly past two women walking along the road with the help of wheeled walkers.

"Check it out, Dad, I can drive!"

Dominic stared ahead and gave a thumbs-up. He was using this gesture a lot now.

Nic drove past the walking women and around the local neighborhood and then ventured onto small, unfamiliar residential roads with multiple speed bumps; he revved over them all fast enough to loosen our teeth.

Stop sign, stop sign.

"I see it, Mom, don't say anything!"

I didn't say a word, but by the end of our ride, I was in need of some of Dominic's medication, and Dominic was as cool as a cucumber.

"Mom's a bit freaked!" said Nic as he walked arm in arm with Dominic back to his room. "At least you think I'm pretty good."

Dom looked ahead and smiled.

Mitch arrived for another visit and walked back to Dominic's room with us. Moments later, there was a soft knock on the door.

"Hello. Can I come in?"

Dominic acknowledged his neighbor with a smile. She lived a few doors up the hall.

"Oh, to see you two dance the other day!" she said.

"I hope the music wasn't too loud?" I said.

"No, not at all."

"How are you?"

"Life is beautiful."

Life was always beautiful for Sister Mary Catherine. She struck me as one of the more serene souls on the planet. She softened the feel of the air we breathed. She walked over to the quilt.

"I've been waiting to see you so I could ask....Can you tell me about this one?" She pointed to the fabric photo of the boys with the words *Happy Mother's Day* painted across their smiling faces. She stroked her hand over the fabric.

"I can feel Dominic's heartbeat in this," she said.

"I like that one, too," said Michael.

"Yeah, that day was really cool. We were much younger then. How old were we?" Nic looked over at Mike.

"Dunno—seven and eight, maybe? We put our heads together so Dad could write the one message with face paint across both of our faces."

They leaned in closer to look at the photo.

"We made Mom breakfast. Dad helped us and we took it to her in bed. I remember she kissed us, and we smeared wet paint all over her face!"

"The breakfast was pretty gross, but Mum ate it anyway and kept offering Dad bites!"

"He kept saying, 'No, it's your special breakfast, it's all for you!'"

Sister Mary Catherine laughed.

After she said goodbye, Dominic got into bed and drifted off to sleep. Although she never popped in for long, she always left her serenity behind.

Mike turned the music down. Nicolas fumbled in Dominic's chest of drawers, looking for the box of fabric pens. He chose a purple one and carefully wrote another inscription around one of Dominic's painted footprints. He put the pen back in its box and pulled a chair up to Dominic's bedside where he sat motionless, watching his father sleep.

A stream of tears ran down his cheeks. He made no attempt to wipe them away. Mitch sat on the floor facing his friend. He leaned calmly against the quilted wall, present: no need to fix, no need to talk.

That night, something woke me. Dominic was standing on a step flanked by four angels. There was so much light: a brilliance impenetrable by dark. He didn't want to leave but he wasn't fighting it either. He cocked his head slightly and smiled at me. There were no words but, when it was time to go, he motioned for the two angels standing closest to me to stay behind. They came and stood with me, one on either side. I felt the brush of their presence on my skin as I sat in my bed, wide awake.

22

The sun rose early, as it does during Brisbane summers. I woke at 6:00 a.m. to the sound of birds singing, with the sun already halfway up the sky.

I hopped out of bed, went to the kitchen to put on the kettle, and walked through to Nic's room to wish him happy birthday. Before I could get to him with a tender motherly kiss, Mike jumped on Nic's bed, ripped off his sheets, and sang out in his radio DJ voice, "Rise 'n' shine!"

Nicolas groaned and put a pillow over his head.

"Happy birthday, sweetheart," I said.

"What time is it?"

"Time to wake up—birthday breakfast coming up soon!" said Mike.

He pulled his brother halfway off the bed by the ankles and left him snoozing—knees on the ground, chest horizontal on the mattress, and a pillow still over his head.

"Don't come out until we are ready!"

Mike closed Nic's door, and he and I went off to prepare the table out on the patio with all the items that form our family birthday breakfast ritual. I moved our homemade Christmas tree, made of attractive dried branches and ornaments, to the dining room table.

We had celebrated Christmas three days ago with a more traditional tree in Dom's room.

I reboiled the kettle. Michael brought out the crockery. I got fresh cuttings from the garden and heard more clattering in the kitchen.

"Hey, Mum? Where's the life candle?"

"In the cupboard."

"Which cupboard?"

"The one it's always in."

"Which one's that?"

There was last-minute wrapping, some finger-licking of cake topping, and lighting of candles. When everything was ready, Michael went to the kitchen, grabbed hold of a dishcloth, and made his way toward Nic's room.

"What about one of my nice scarves?"

"Nah, this'll be fine."

"Egh! This one is rank!" said Nic as Mike blindfolded him.

The blindfold ritual had become more and more boyish over the last few years. My colorful scarves had long been discarded for damp dishcloths or smelly sports socks.

Michael proceeded to take his blindfolded brother on a round-about journey toward the breakfast table while I followed with my camera. When he reached the table, he spun Nic around until he was dizzy before removing the blindfold. Birthday splendor and a happy birthday song greeted Nic. His placemat was decorated with flowers from the garden. Next to it stood his life candle with a strong flame. There were sparklers, our homemade card sitting amongst cards that had arrived from overseas, a few gifts, hot tea served from an old bone china tea set given to my parents on their engagement, and, on this particular morning, a massive pavlova dripping with fruit and cream. Cake of your choice for breakfast—it was the highlight of birthdays when the boys were younger and, despite finding it less appealing to eat cake this early in the day now that the boys were older, no one wanted to lose this part of the tradition.

We sat around the table getting high on sugar and cream washed down with tea.

"I dare you to eat a whole pavlova in one go."

"How much?"

"Ten bucks."

"Ten?!"

"Okay, fifteen."

"Deal."

"Why would you do that? You'll get sick," I said.

Nic smiled. He took a moment, gathered a wish for his life, and breathed it silently out into the world as he blew out his life candle.

When breakfast was over, we packed some pavlova into a container and drove out to McCorely. We celebrated Nic's birthday again with Dominic. He had a few spoonfuls of the sweet meringue despite not being able to taste it.

"Hey, Dad, you reckon I could eat a whole pav in one go?"

Dominic smiled.

He was becoming increasingly frail. I had the sense of Death waiting patiently in the wings. I pleaded with it to wait a bit longer. *Please, not today, not on Nic's birthday.*

A nurse popped her head in, wished Nic happy birthday, and asked if she could see me. When I got back to Dominic's room, he had dozed off. The boys and I drove home, leaving him to rest.

I wrote to my family later that same afternoon.

I have to go to the funeral home tomorrow to look at coffins. One of the nurses spoke to me today and said I should do it now rather than wait. They do a special goodbye here when a body leaves their care, but I didn't know I had to prearrange anything. What can I say? I wasn't really prepared for that conversation today. It's Nic's birthday, my friends are out buying new summer shoes at the Boxing Day sales, and I'm heading out to buy a coffin. It's one of those days where everything and nothing makes sense.

Nic's friends arrived and kicked off the evening with a comical attempt at a game of poker. This small gathering of close friends sat themselves around the dining room table all dressed up for the show. Mitch dimmed the lights, pulled his hoodie up over his head, and dealt the cards. The clink of plastic chips and the sound of munching—lots and lots of munching—interrupted the quietness. They all made their best possible hands. Eight poker faces stared at each other from behind an array of dark glasses, each of them trying to get a read on his opponents. Someone raised and then scratched his head under an annoying straw hat that was way too small. Nic called and pulled a large, floppy beach hat down over his face. If it weren't for the hilarious assortment of hats these boys wore to try and hide their facial expressions, it would have looked like an underground gangster gathering, as if at any moment they'd be busting out cigars.

Hands moved repetitively from bowls to mouths, and losers slowly migrated to the couch in front of the PlayStation where they played Madden and munched some more. I woke the next morning to sleeping bodies stretched out and snoring in the family room. No one stirred when the phone rang. It was Patricia, checking in.

"What are you up to today?" she said.

"I have to go to the funeral place to choose a coffin."

"What? Who's going with you?"

"No one. I'll be fine."

"You shouldn't have to do that alone. Can I come with you?"

"I'll be fine, really."

"You won't know that until you walk in there. I'm coming with you."

The funeral director greeted us warmly; she knew the McCorely ritual well. I stood before the selection of empty coffins, lined in satin, all waiting for Dominic.

A whisper lurched up from my insides. "What am I doing here? He's not even dead yet."

Patricia took my hand and squeezed. The funeral director blinked back tears. I stood there, choking, floating, breathing; slowly breathing until the emptiness found a way to settle and just was. When the silence had held me, I chose the one on the left.

"Dominic would want something simple," I said.

23

Dominic made it through Nic's birthday. Then came New Year's Eve, and he was the best he had been in a while. I took him for a drive to Nudgee Beach. We sat together on a bench overlooking the water at low tide. Two black Labradors chased each other in and out of the water as they ran along the sand flats.

"Want an ice cream?"

Dominic shook his head. He sat motionless with a hand on each knee, the urge to pace momentarily eased. He stared across the bay to Stradbroke Island. We sat like this until his legs started to jiggle and the agitated desire to move returned. He stood up. Arms hanging by his sides, he shuffled back to the car. I took him for another drive. His legs jiggled like a jammed-up toy with no off switch, but the rhythm of the moving car helped the rest of him be still. He looked straight ahead beyond the life around him; past the fishermen, the mangroves, and a group of cyclists riding the same bike path we had ridden as a family in another lifetime.

I drove on, taking the long way round, hoping it would soothe him, before slowly making my way back to the nursing home.

I climbed into bed with him that night. He touched my hand and rested his crackling head on my chest, his body giving way to sleep and relaxing into softness, until restless leg movement possessed him once again and the plastic undersheet rustled. I looked at his sleeping face tilted toward mine. How much longer did we have?

Maybe if I imagined he was dead, I could prepare. Maybe if I did that, I would be able to let him go. Maybe I could stave off the dread. Maybe I would be able to face driving home one day knowing I'd never again feel his body against mine.

So, I stared at him. He was a body. He was gone. The goneness throttled me. My heart clambered around, urgently looking for him, until I felt the body in my arms breathe lightly on my face. His breath stroked me as I closed my eyes and went to the place in my heart where I was storing him. I felt his warmth and inhaled the breath that escaped him, absorbing him, so that when he was gone, there would always be a part of me that could feel him.

I drifted into a dream. We were kayaking somewhere. The sky was full of cockatoos, golden eagles, and butterflies. Dominic leaned his tired body against my back, and we floated into the timeless wisdom of nature.

I followed the eagles and paddled to the edge of the world.

The sound of my vibrating phone on the bedside table steered me back to the nursing home. I woke to see Liz's name lit up on the display.

"Sorry, did I wake you?"

"It's okay. I need to go home to the boys anyway."

"Is 8:00 a.m. too early for our walk tomorrow?"

"No, it's perfect."

"Great, see you then."

I slid my arm out from under Dominic's sleeping head and slipped out of his bed. I stood by his side and watched his skeletal body breathe, unconsciously twisting my wedding ring around and around my finger.

Please, if I'm doing anything that is holding Dominic here, help me to let him go.

I kissed him and walked out, one foot in front of the other, down the corridor of shiny clean floors, through the quiet of nighttime sleeping and the padded footsteps of a night nurse doing her rounds, past the nurses' station, through the dimmed lighting of the entrance foyer, and out of the main doors into the night air of the outside world.

Liz and Ed often "walked me" before I drove out to the nursing home each morning. I met them as planned at 8:00 a.m. We passed a few joggers on the bike path when I felt a painful stab on my finger.

"Ouch!"

"What's wrong?" asked Liz.

I looked at my left hand. My wedding ring had snapped and was pinching my skin. It was a simple, three-band Russian wedding ring, and all three bands had snapped right through in one clean slice.

"How on earth did that happen?" she said.

I have to take it off?

"You'll have to take it off."

I fiddled with it, trying to find a way to keep it on, but it wasn't going to hold.

"You'll lose it. You need to take it off. Here, give it to me. I have a pocket."

"No, it's okay," I said, holding on to it.

Clasping a lifetime in my palm, I finished the walk. The shops were all closed, but I was the first person at the jeweler when stores reopened after the New Year public holiday. The assistant at the counter had a look at it.

"We should have it ready in about two weeks," she said.

"Is there any chance it can be done before then? Please, it's really important." *My husband is dying. I don't think we have two weeks.*

The jeweler was off sick. He had several jobs waiting, but she would put it in as a priority, she said. They would get to it as soon as they could.

My phone rang.

"Hey, sis." It was Reagen calling from San Diego.

"Hi."

"Are you okay?"

"I don't know."

"It's just…I saw Dominic last night."

"You saw him?"

"It was the middle of the night, and I got up to go to the bathroom. When I came back to bed he was standing right in front of me. Marie, I was wide awake. He didn't say anything, but he smiled."

"And then?"

"I thought I was imagining things, so I closed my eyes and opened them again and he was still there. Then he disappeared. I wanted to check if you were okay."

I drove out to Dominic that morning, holding Reagen's vision in my mind. My bare ring finger felt odd against the steering wheel. I walked into Dominic's room, past the life that smiled at me from the fabric wall, and sat on his bed. He saw me and gave that familiar crooked smile.

He was fully aware. I saw it in the look behind his tear-brimmed eyes.

He leaned into my hold. I got the sense he was saying he wasn't ready to go, that there was still so much he wanted to share with us, but that he was letting go. He couldn't control this. He shifted his body and wrapped his thin arms around me.

"Are you scared?"

"No," he whispered into my neck. I felt the wetness of his tears. I could taste them. He sat back against his pillow. "I'm just so…sad."

And then he drifted away—back inside with the Green Goblin. Both our eyes were still wet. We spent the day together, in and out of words, awareness, and confusion; the nothingness, the fullness, the pacing, trees blowing, Stradbroke calling. And like most of my evenings, I went home to the boys when he was fast asleep.

The phone woke me in the early hours of the next morning. Dominic was failing, the nurse on night duty explained; we were called in. We arrived just as the sun began to warm the sky. Dominic lay on his back, very still. I went to his side and gently stroked his arm.

"Hi, Dom. We're all here. Look, your two boys are here."

He slowly opened his eyes, forcing the weight of the drugs from his eyelids. The boys moved to flank him: one on each side of the bed.

He looked from one son to the other. A smile spread itself magically over the rigidity that had claimed his face. He reached out and took hold of their hands and brought them in over his heart.

"My…two…boys…are…here."

He closed his eyes, and lay with their hands clasped to his chest.

Slowly breathing in and out.

Breathing, not breathing.

Breathing.

Hands relaxing.

Sleeping.

After some time, Michael walked over to the quilt. He pulled the lid off a fabric pen with his teeth and left it in his mouth as he wrote around Dominic's footprints—bold writing with blue twirls drawn above and below his message.

The day rolled on, and the boys lay on their mattresses on the floor, sending out texts. Their phones beeped with multiple replies.

"What's with all the texting?"

"We weren't going to tell you 'cause it was supposed to be a surprise. We planned a surprise birthday party for you at Felicity's tonight—we're just cancelling it."

I looked at them, stunned.

"We managed to steal most of the numbers from your phone."

"You guys are amazing!" I sat on the mattress with them. "Seriously amazing."

"Nah, we wanted something nice for you. And, anyway, Felicity's been doing all the hard work."

"I love you guys. I really love you."

"Well, it's just on hold. Genevieve and Felicity are calling everyone for us now, but we'll still do something sometime. It's just...we don't know when..." said Mike.

"I don't want Dad to die on your birthday," said Nic.

"I'll be okay."

"I know you, you'll go and make something all meaningful out of it, but still, I think it would be horrible."

I ruffled his hair. He tried to duck.

"And, anyway, I know you didn't want Dad to die on my birthday."

I looked out of the window. Evening shadows crept across the lawn as the sky was slowly drained of light.

There was reading, checking for breath, touching, a game of chess, a few jokes, laughter, and chitchat until the shadows lurched into the room and landed on the boys' chests.

"This waiting is intense, Mum," said Michael from a hollow face. "I don't think I can stay the night."

"You okay?"

"I need to get out of here. I want to go home."

"But there's no one at home."

"I'll stay at Jack's. This waiting is doing my head in."

He walked over to Dominic, leaned over him, and whispered, "I love you, Dad."

Dominic opened his eyes. "I love you, Mike."

Michael's kiss landed with the gentleness of a butterfly. He looked back up at me. His eyes were as soft as his voice. "I can go now."

Nic watched.

"What do you want to do?" I asked him.

"I want to stay. But don't leave me alone with Dad."

"Sweetheart, you don't have to stay."

"I want to. I need to."

I turned to Mike. "Promise me you won't be alone."

"Promise."

Felicity and Jack drove out to pick him up.

Nic fell asleep on the mattress on the floor, and I dozed on the bed next to Dominic between the many nursing observations. By morning, Dominic had stabilized.

"Happy birthday, Mom!" said Nic through a morning yawn.

He climbed out of bed and gave me a hug. He looked over at Dominic and back at me.

"He's okay," I said.

Dominic was sleeping restfully.

Nic walked over to the quilt and looked at the image of his dad throwing him up in the air as a toddler. "I want to be like that when I'm a dad."

He ran his hands over the picture as I brushed my teeth. I imagined how Dom would feel hearing those words.

After checking in with the nurses, we left early, before Dominic woke, and drove home. I was immediately relegated to my bedroom while the boys prepared a birthday breakfast: garden flowers on my placemat, a life candle, tea poured from the same bone china teapot into delicate teacups—their saucers delightfully forgotten and still sitting in the kitchen cupboard. There was a chocolate mud cake from The Cheesecake Shop topped with chocolate-dipped profiteroles, a card drawn with ballpoint pen and fluorescent highlighters on paper whipped out of the printer tray, and a soft silk scarf as a blindfold.

"It's your birthday!" said Dominic when we returned to McCorely later that afternoon. Where did he find those words? And how did he know?

I hadn't said anything. He beamed a smile. These moments of clarity were precious, a bundling together of simple life treasures before they were lost again.

Beth was there, sitting cross-legged on the adjoining bed, decorating a new door sign with Dominic's name on it. She had spent the morning quietly singing with him as they paced, or massaging his hands and feet. For much of the time, she was simply there. She understood the value of stillness, the richness in being, and the gift of doing nothing.

Dominic was so much better that day, despite his agitated pacing, and when the evening arrived, he was unusually relaxed. The Green Goblin was quiet; it seemed to be giving him a break. His sleep was tranquil and silent. We were used to the breathy rattle. Nic looked at his chest to make sure it was moving. Mike put his cheek over Dominic's slightly open mouth, feeling for breath. Their faces relaxed.

The two hospital beds were pushed together to create a double bed. Careful not to disturb Dominic's sleep, the three of us lay squished on the one mattress. We ate junk food and watched *Walk the Line* so that if Dominic woke he could enjoy the music of Johnny Cash without having to understand the story.

"Dude, I'm falling off here."

"I can't help it."

"Lie on your side or something."

"Uh—no! So now we all gonna spoon?"

"Dude! Just lie on your side. It'll make more room."

"I think I need to stretch." Nic stretched his arms and legs over me and across to Michael on the other side of the bed. "This feels gooood."

"Dickhead!"

Nic snatched the bag of chips from Michael's hands. Chips scattered amongst the laughter and fell on us like autumn leaves shaken from a salty sky. My phone beeped over the banter: a text from Genevieve.

Can I visit?

Love that.

Am right outside your door.

I climbed over the boys, who immediately filled the spare space.

I opened the door to a bunch of flowers.

"Happy birthday, honey!" She carried in an additional vase of pink roses sent from friends in Canada and popped them on the table.

"He looks so peaceful," she said. She took Dominic's pulse and gently stroked his hair. I left the boys to finish the chips while Genevieve and I went out to the kitchenette.

"How are you doing?"

"Okay about not being okay..."

This had become my standard response.

She popped a tea bag each into two mugs and filled them from the boiling water tap.

"Nic is very pale. Please don't stay tonight. Take both boys home," she said as she poured.

"He's pale?"

"He really is. I see the strain all over his face."

"Sometimes I don't know what to do....Should we stay, should we go? What if..."

"Nic did what he needed to do; he stayed last night. But now I think he needs you to take him home. When he is here, he follows you everywhere, he won't leave your side. Right now, he needs to be with you, not with Dominic."

Mike came out into the corridor to answer his phone and, as if on cue, Nicolas came into the kitchenette to find me.

"Tea, sweetheart?"

"No, thanks."

I casually put my arm around him. He moved in closer. He didn't want to be the only one with Dominic. What if Dominic died when he was alone with him?

With my arm still around Nic, I looked around the kitchen of what had become my second home. Only nine weeks ago I had driven Dom out here for his respite stay, knowing he would not come home. I realized I had a different sense of place here than the boys. People here were witness to a part of our story no one else could see; it gave me somewhere solid to stand in this disintegrating life. In turn, I heard stories from this new community of people I had been invited to join—stories of forbidden love, yearnings to go home, child-care problems, cycling adventures, grieving hearts, and the desire to work Christmas shifts to escape family drama at home.

I gave Nic a squeeze, then checked on Dom, who was still asleep, and took the boys home. They spent much of the car ride texting, but I paid no attention—find me one teenager who doesn't send multiple messages from phones transformed in puberty into vital organs. Two minutes after we arrived home, Felicity, Christian, and their whole family entourage arrived. They followed Felicity, holding a birthday cake alight with candles, through the front door and out onto our patio.

"See?" said Michael, eyebrows raised and smiling. "The benefits of texting!"

Felicity's daughter-in-law, a trained opera singer, burst into an operatic version of "Happy Birthday." Our neighbors on the other side had people over for dinner. They stopped to listen as her voice rang out into the quiet night sky.

I woke the next day before the morning light and sat up in bed. Something was different. I had to get back to the nursing home. I arrived early and alone as Dom woke to a day of struggle.

As the day wore on, I saw some nurses cry. None of Dom's medicines were working.

The garden-boot doctor took me to another room where we could talk. There was a new drug that might help. Dominic would go into a deep sleep and lose awareness of his suffering. He needed my consent. The doctor held my hand as I agreed. It might make it easier for Dom to let go.

I held Dominic's hand and stroked his head as the drug was added to the cocktail already being fed into his body. His hand lay limp in mine but his legs twitched with urgency: the Green Goblin was still desperate to move. In and out of bed. In and out of bed.

"Feet..." Dom said.

I massaged his feet, sending love toward his heart, hoping he would feel it.

The nurse left us alone together.

I wet his lips with a sponge and stroked his contorted body, trying not to hear the rattling gasps from which he was detaching. We lay there together on the edge of life.

Would he understand my whisperings to let go? He was fighting this. How could I gently take him there?

"Let's go to Straddie, Dom."

He nodded.

I held him as he followed my prompts.

Together, we went to the island. He allowed the warmth of the sun to caress his skin; he put his face toward the wind and let it blow through his hair. He felt the sand between his toes. Sunshine scattered glitter on the waves that were calling. He took my hand and walked with me toward the sea. Weightless, he entered the water. The ocean held him as he opened his eyes one last time.

"I...love...you...Marie."

"I love you, too, Dom."

"I know..."

In and out of sleep.

Chest rattling; waves rolling; safely falling.

Slipping deeper; water rising; lungs filling.

I heard the clip-clop of shoes. *Maggie?* It was a Saturday but she had come in.

"He sounds terrible," I said.

"It's worse for you than it is for him. He can't feel this." She held his hand. I stroked his head. "I'll stay with him. Why don't you go home and get some sleep?"

"How can I leave him like this?"

Exhaustion had attached itself to me, but was so familiar I didn't feel it. I heard her reassuring voice and something about being no good to anyone if I was exhausted. She gently urged me to go home and get some sleep so that I could have some reserves to face what was to come.

I wanted to lean on her and cry, cry my eyes out, but I held on to the bed rails and felt the cold bars hold me together like a splint.

The doctor told me Dominic's heart was still strong and his color was good. He was young, with strong organs; he thought it would be another couple of days before his system would shut down.

I leaned over Dominic and whispered to him through the water in which he was floating. I kissed his hollow cheek, and as I slipped my hand out of his, Maggie stepped in to stroke his head and talk softly to him. I left the room, walking backward, watching frailty held so safely within tenderness. He wasn't alone; I knew he could hear her.

I called the boys from the car. They were still out with Mitch and Jack, so I went home via Genevieve's.

"Honey, you are completely dehydrated," she said before I had even said hello.

She sat me down on a chair on her back deck, fed and watered me, and listened. The twins came and went, curling up in my lap and dosing me with affection that was pure and unafraid. I checked in with Maggie. Dominic had been given his next dose of the new drug. He was settled and in no pain. With that reassurance, I drove home, but only after promising Genevieve I would not drive out there that night. I was too tired, it wasn't safe, she said. If I was called back in, she would drive me herself.

I opened my front door to a ringing phone. Maggie's voice was calmer than usual.

"Marie, it's Maggie."

I waited.

"Things have taken a turn. I think you should come back."

I don't remember what I said.

"I've told Dominic I am calling you—he knows you are coming."

The boys were still out. I tried to call them, but the calls went to voicemail. I tried again; same thing. I called Genevieve, still holding my keys, as I flew to the car.

I felt the moment Dominic left this earth. My back wheels met the road as I reversed out of the driveway. I looked up to the sky as if I might see him. I felt his exhaustion, the kind that needs holding and is coupled with relief after taking the step of which he had been most frightened: letting go.

Dom!

Genevieve was waiting for me in her driveway. I parked and ran to her car.

"He's gone, Gen," I said as she pulled off.

She reached for my hand.

We drove the rest of the way in silence.

Maggie was waiting for us at the main entrance at McCorely. There could be only one reason she was waiting for us there. I fell into her arms as she told me what I already knew. A hollow sound groaned from my chest and tumbled down the long, empty corridors until it fell over Dominic. Every facet of grief I had left hanging outside the front door of McCorely these past weeks followed me into his room that night.

I crumpled over him, my unstoppable tears washing his cooling body.

His jaw drooped and his mouth lay open. The room swirled. I wished his mouth was closed.

I held him a while as he lay openmouthed, finally dead after slowly dying. But he was still there somehow, as if he had died without really leaving.

Dominic had died holding Maggie's hand and, despite the vigil I had kept, I did not get there in time. There would be months and months ahead of me feeling I had failed him. I wasn't there. Why did I go home? I had intuited so many things before—how did I not know he was finally leaving? Perhaps, in choosing his moment to die, he had looked after us all, and he still had a say. Did he try to spare me?

But why? I was excluded from this ultimate intimacy; he chose someone else.

In time, I would wonder how hard it might have been for him to die with us all gathered around him. The intensity and sadness as we waited for this dreaded event might have made it harder for him to let go. Perhaps my leaving released him? In some way, we both departed. But, most of all, when I could bear to be honest enough, could I forgive myself for being relieved that I had been spared?

The boys. I had to tell the boys. I squeezed Dominic's dead hand, noticed his crinkled sheets, and felt Genevieve stroke my hair. This was no phone conversation. Genevieve drove me home to get them.

"So, what's your most annoying memory of Dominic?" she asked in the car.

"He used to sneak into the bathroom and throw cold water over me in the shower. It drove me nuts!" I chortled through waves of dizziness.

It was a game he and his two brothers had played as kids. Dominic and the boys did it to each other, too. They all found this prank much funnier than I ever did. I got Dominic back plenty of times, but it wasn't nearly as satisfying when I knew this absolutely guaranteed I would be doused again.

The boys weren't home when Genevieve and I got there. What is the best way to tell your sons their dad has died when they are out with friends? Mike was with Jack, driving Jack's sister back from a party. Nic was at Mitch's house with a few friends. He would be there for a while.

I waited for Mike to come home. I started moving things around on my dresser: the paperweight Mike had made for me when he was little—a large, smooth river stone with a faded painted face and paper headdress; a Rubik's cube, the one Dominic used to crack; a blue ceramic pig Nic had made, with curly ears and a Manchester United logo down its back. It felt like forever, but I didn't have to wait more than five minutes for Mike to come home. We sat together on my bed. I saw sadness flutter across his face. We went to Mitch's house to get Nic. There was no reason for me to knock on the door so late at night other than to tell him his dad had died. When Mike and I came to the door, he simply picked up his backpack, left his friends without saying a word, and came outside.

I told him as we sat on a garden bench on Mitch's patio.

Genevieve was parked in the road under a streetlamp, waiting for us as long as we needed before driving us back to McCorely. When we were all in the car, I turned to face the backseat. Both boys looked a hundred years old.

We pulled into the parking lot. There was no need to hide the car around the back; Dominic wouldn't try to follow us home tonight. We went to his room. He was surrounded by family photos and the fresh flowers we always had on his bedside table. He was now tucked into a neatly made bed with his arms out over the sheets and his hands clasped over his chest holding an angel. The spare beds had been moved out of the room. Nobody lived here anymore.

A draft blew us the touch of a lover's kiss and a father's pull toward his sons; a desperate hope they could hear him saying their names; a sudden burst of energy and an invitation to play soccer or one last game of chess before a sad stillness as he watched his boys walk toward his body.

"He's so cold…" said Mike.

The boys ran their hands across his face. They felt over his mouth for the possibility of breath. They put their cheeks against his and stroked his paper-thin skin.

They took off his medic-alert bracelet. Michael held it up. *Frontotemporal Dementia with ALS—contact wife Marie*, followed by our phone number.

We placed his tiny silver angel on his pillow and added a rose to his hands.

We nibbled on biscuits and sipped on the overly sweet lemonade left for us in the room.

We wept. We talked. We sat in that quiet space where both love and loss were finely sensed. I don't know how long we were there.

I looked at our two boys. "Would you like some time alone with Dad?"

Nic nodded. We tucked Dom into bed one last time and, kissing him, Mike and I said goodbye and left the room.

Genevieve drove the three of us home in a silent car through a world that kept on living—cars driving places, people chatting in the glow of buzzing restaurants, lights turning off in bedroom windows as loved ones kissed each other goodnight. The world around me started disappearing, swirling.

Stay here, breathe, just breathe.

Genevieve pulled into our driveway. I walked through our front door and stumbled through to my bedroom.

NO! Not now…the boys have just lost their dad…not now…

Everything went dark. Endless falling.

"Marie, can you hear me?"

"Is Mom okay?"

"She'll be fine," said Genevieve, feeling my pulse. "She's exhausted, and she's feeling it all now because she can. Don't worry. I'll stay here with her."

The boys—get back there to my boys.

In and out of darkness.

"Mike? Nic?"

"You okay, Mom?" I saw the two of them at the end of my bed.

"Do you want to bring mattresses in here? You don't have to sleep alone tonight," I said.

"No, it's okay." They looked at each other.

"She'll be all right," said Genevieve.

Their strong and present mother lay broken open; my raw grief offered them no comfort.

Genevieve climbed into bed with me that night.

"I'm here," she said as she stroked my back, and I sobbed in my sleep.

In the morning, Genevieve brought me a cup of tea and made me drink it. "Here's a piece of toast."

"I don't feel like eating."

"Just a few bites, you have nothing in you."

She watched me nibble and waited for me to finish my tea.

"I'm going to pop home quickly to get some clean clothes and check in on the girls," she said. "The boys are just getting up. They're doing okay. I'll be back in an hour to drive you to McCorely."

"Gen?" She looked over at me. "Thank you…"

She smiled. "Hop into the shower before the boys use up all the hot water!"

She blew me a kiss and let herself out the front door.

The days and weeks to follow would be filled with family and friends from both near and far. Flowers would lean out of vases in beautiful arrangements all through the house. Our home would smell like a florist's, and we would run out of space.

We would pack up Dominic's room. Sister Patricia would pop in. During a moment alone together, she would sit on the bed with me and burst into tears.

"When this is all over," she would say, "let's go away together and get drunk!"

The two of us would screech with laughter and people in earshot would wonder what hilarity had been set off in Dominic's room.

There would be a funeral the next week. The jeweler would ring just as we were leaving for the church to tell me my wedding ring was ready for pickup and that they would be closing at 5:00 p.m. Genevieve's husband would drive us all to the church. My sister's fingers would get slammed in the car door. They would turn blue and swell like sausages in front of us. We would all get back out of the car.

"Let's get some ice."

"No, let's go," she would say to my brother.

"I think we should ice it."

"Just go! C'mon, let's go."

Hundreds of people would turn up, and it would take us by surprise. The quilt would be draped over Dominic's coffin, and I would tuck him in one last time. The boys would join in carrying their dad out of the church and people would weep. They could feel the touch of love, they would say. They would talk about this funeral for a long time.

A few days after the funeral, we would go to the place Dominic had loved and scatter his ashes into the ocean at dawn. The waves would embrace him, my man of the sea. We would stand there a while, watching the sun lift its head from under the world and listening to the sound of the sea. Later that afternoon, the boys would run into the water and bodysurf while the mixture of salt and sand scuffed sadness from their skin. I'd be on the beach watching. I would notice a mother sitting on the rocks keeping an eye on her two little boys boogie boarding in the surf with their dad. I would wonder who was having more fun, the boys or their father.

I would look again—the bowler-hat doctor?! He wouldn't see me and I would wonder if he had any idea Dominic had even died. I would feel Dominic take my left hand. He would walk me away from the world of illness and doctors and take me to the spots we had once lain, lovers entwined and filling up with stars that poured into us from the Stradbroke night. We would linger there together before he splashed me playfully and disappeared back into the sea.

These days and weeks still lay ahead, and while time would unfold with some sense of routine—dinner follows lunch, lunch follows breakfast—grief tends to change the shape of things. Time becomes more elastic, pulling you in and out, a bit like tides of the sea.

For now, however, I had to get ready for the first of these shared rituals that mark death and honor life. I did as Genevieve said.

I hopped into the shower. As the warm water spilled over me, I suddenly, felt it—that mischievous presence that came before a familiar cold water splash.

"Dominic?!"

I instinctively dodged the cold water. Then he left. He was playing! Was he telling me he was okay? I started to laugh. *Oh God, how can I laugh? He just died.* And then I cried. I leaned against the shower wall and let the running water wash a mixture of laughter and tears from me.

I heard the phone ring. I grabbed a towel and wrapped it around me, holding it with one hand as I answered the phone in the bedroom, still soaking wet.

"Hello, Mrs. Williams," said a friendly female voice from the funeral home. "Could you please tell us if your husband was tall? We want to make sure we bring out the right size coffin to McCorely."

I watched my two big soggy footprints expand on the carpet.

"Yes...he was tall."

I got dressed and heard the clatter of breakfast dishes in the kitchen. The boys were as pale as the walls. I gave them both a hug.

"How did you sleep last night?"

"Fine," said Mike.

I looked at Nic.

"Fine…" He scraped his bowl. "We're fine, Mom." *Stop asking us.* "How 'bout you? Did you sleep?"

"Sort of."

He added his empty bowl to the sink full of dishes, filled it with water, and left it soaking.

"I don't think I want to go back into Dad's room," said Nic.

"Me either," said Mike.

"None of us have to."

"I said goodbye already." It was Nic who said it, but I knew it was how they both felt. "So many times. I can't do it over and over and over again."

Genevieve drove us to McCorely. Jack came along in the car. Beth was already there when we arrived. So were Sister Patricia, Liz, Ed, and their teenage children. They had already been with Dom and gathered around us as friends, coresidents, and staff dropped in to see Dominic with a kiss, a private conversation, a flower. Sometime later the funeral directors arrived with the coffin I had chosen: big enough for a tall person. They walked past us all. I watched the coffin trolley turn the corner and enter his room.

Maggie helped them place Dominic's body inside the simple wooden box. She led him, lying in his quilt-covered coffin, out of his room and down the corridor. The familiar clip-clop of her shoes tapped through the hallway and then stopped. She paused, wiped her eyes with a tissue, and then lifted her head. She took a deep breath and walked with Dom toward us.

A resident, wearing thick, rubber-soled shoes, banged her wheeled walker into the back of another's wheelchair. She was oblivious to the clang that echoed through the silence and the scowl thrown back at her from the silver-haired woman with milky eyes. I slipped my hands into the boys' and felt Liz's touch on my shoulder. A guard of honor formed as Dominic came through to us. Patricia watched me from across the room through unblinked tears, and Genevieve whispered something into Beth's ear. One voice in the crowd started to sing—a voice graced with the wobble of age. A chorus of voices joined her singing in Latin. The sound grew.

"*Salve, Regina, Mater misericordiae,*
Vita, dulcedo, et spes nostra, salve…"

The nuns were used to singing together, a familiar unity of voices, harmonizing and absorbing the tones of anyone off-key. The hymn, known in English as "Hail Holy Queen," rose on their breath, filling the room. Dominic always had a thing for Mary.

"Strong mind, gentle heart," he would say about her.

His "life motto," he called it. It went back to his high school days.

Voices sang in communal song, holding us.

"*O clemens, O pia, O dulcis Virgo Maria.*"

I stood in the sound, lost yet acutely present.

The boys and I accompanied our strong and gentle Dominic out of the building. The singing procession followed us outside.

Voices lifting. Breathing out to let breath in. Singing beyond the sky.

The quilt flapped in the breeze as the coffin slid into the hearse.

We watched the long silver car slowly drive out of sight.

Dominic rested quietly on the other side of my breath.

"Let's go home, Mom," said Nic. He put his arm around me. "It's done."

Epilogue

It's a strange thing, weaving together threads of the past from a place in the present. I've written a story about us, but I am not quite the same person I was back then.

I have been to the place where heaven and earth meet; that liminal space where time does not exist, only love calling us to our fullest potential. In balancing the deep, otherworldly experience of grief with the material world I am called back into, I can look back and see that in Dominic's unraveling, he spiraled me into something new. We are all different now.

This story is about a particular time in our life, but I wish for it to be bigger than that. It is a story of love and life. A tale of a strange place—the real world—in which green goblins and hope find a way to live together.

It was originally written with no intention of publication. My writing started out as a spontaneous, creative response to grief with no thought of placing this part of our life on display: this menacing creature, monstrous and vague; the strange ways; our blended beloved who was slowly lost.

By the time Dominic was diagnosed, he had already been robbed of so much, and I was no longer able to share conversations with him as we had before. I started to write emails to special people in my life who were able to listen and join us on a journey that might otherwise have been very lonely. We were fairly new immigrants to Australia. Very few people around us knew the fullness of the Dominic we had known. I found myself writing emails to family and trusted friends overseas with whom I had shared long and significant histories. They knew us as a close family; they had known and loved Dominic as a well man; and they anchored me to a shared reality we had all once lived together.

After Dominic died and insomnia rolled my days and nights into one, I wrote even more. I felt the connection of this scattered community. My family and friends received my raw and unvarnished thoughts in real time and, despite their physical distance, I felt closely held by them.

Looking back, I can see how writing provided refuge from the chaos, a safe haven for reflection where I could try and make sense of my changing world. It gave me time to pause, to notice when the space between life and death, between being and not being, felt profoundly sacred. It held still the paradox, where life was both empty and full, together and falling apart, and the simplest things were the most extraordinary. It was a way to outstare the darkness, and it became an act of advocacy. Dominic had lost his speech, but he was not voiceless. He was held hostage by this illness and stripped of almost everything, but he was so much more than his circumstances. And as Dominic got sicker, it helped me to challenge the ideas our culture upholds about what it means to be a contributing and valued participant in our society.

Recipients of my emails encouraged me to write our story. My brother said he had saved every email I had written. Without knowing it, perhaps this book was already writing itself. However, the deciding factor in collating my musings was a request from Michael and Nicolas. Dominic had been gone about eighteen months. They came to me within one week of each other, following separate experiences with friends that had left them feeling the alienation of disenfranchised grief.

Michael had been out with a group of friends. I think it was one of the Jackie Chan films that lost the toss of movie choice and they settled in to watch *The Notebook*, a love story about an older couple where the narrator's partner has dementia. There were lots of tears. Michael was comforted by the emotional response evoked by this "chick flick," but he felt simultaneously invalidated by the lack of connection his friends made to his own story with dementia. He was a teenager. His dad had been a young man, younger even than many of his friends' dads. There was absolutely no place for him to fit into this narrative. His experience of love and loss with dementia felt imperceptible. He stood alone in this landscape and came home that night feeling erased. Knowing others had asked me to do so, he asked me to write about what we had lived, "to give the story form."

One week later, Nic opened up to a friend who had not known him well during Dominic's illness. His friend was a warm and compassionate listener, but Nic had felt things he could not describe. His experience lay somewhere beyond articulation. Like Michael, it left him straddling two separate realms with no bridge between the two: the one where his story was lived and felt, and the other where there were no words to make it real to others. He came home that night, not knowing Michael had spoken to me the week before, and he, too, asked me to write about it, "to try and capture it somehow."

The three of us talked together about how difficult it was to express the madness of our lives back then from a place of calm. The contradiction was silencing. It had been a life-shaping experience, but it was not a tangible concept. It was confusing but very real. It was powerful, dismantling, and strange. So much of what we lived had bolted past us in chaotic haste. It was slippery, invisible, and wordless. I asked if they would like to write this story with me. We could write it just for us and then we could see how we felt.

While the boys have chosen not to write here, they have been involved in every evolving chapter and their words are scattered throughout the book. My writing of *Green Vanilla Tea* became the launching pad for wondrously rich conversations with them and, with their permission, many of their reflections and thoughts have been captured here, giving the story form. What I have written is by nature only part of a story. It has to be. It is impossible to compress all the complexities of this particular time in our lives into one book, let alone the richness of life lived alongside it, and, as the writer, my voice is automatically privileged. It is a story shaped by my (and the boys') memories. Like the quilt that helped us reconstruct meaning while Dominic was alive, writing this book became a vehicle through which we started healing after he had died. Slowly, we found a way to describe some of what we experienced in all its disheveled fluctuations.

Outside the world of biomedical language, which clarifies pertinent symptoms and options for treatment, there is no social discourse for understanding frontotemporal lobar dementia in a young person—not that we found, anyway. And Dom had amyotrophic lateral sclerosis along with it. He had the two damn wretched things together. At the time we were living this, there were no established services for young people, no common language to help convey or understand the multiple needs of a family in this situation. There were no stories, no clues. People associate the word "chemo" with cancer; there are pink ribbons and bandanas. There are no such ready-made signifiers for teens who have a young parent with FTD ALS. There are no books or movies about it; there are no "We Are the World"–type songs or "Shave for a Cure" community drives. We understood there would probably never be an awareness ribbon for the likes of us, and, even if there was, would we wear one? Probably not. But in a social context, without signifiers of any kind, where does your experience go? How does one talk about it? Is it even real?

The way we use words is important, but it is more than a vehicle for understanding things; it has a profound effect on how we experience ourselves. Discourses affect the shape of life. No wonder Mike and Nic felt invisible. We knew of no one else in our shoes, no one walking our story. Yet, as Christina Baldwin says in her book *Storycatcher*, stories that are shared have the power to create connection, to establish community, and to provide us with the opportunity to recognize ourselves in each other's lives. This is what we were missing.

In *The Australian PhotoJournalist: Picturing Human Rights*, David Lloyd says that stories, when voiced, become a political act. "It doesn't change the world, but storytelling changes people and people change the world." Telling this story is for us as much a political act as it is a story of love and hope.

So, filled with paradox and discovery, I wrote. In the company of hot tea, cupping my hands around the mug and watching the steam rise, I tried once more to capture my thoughts before they evaporated.

Writing in silence, but not alone.

This is for my boys.

Bibliography

Andreas, Brian. *Living Memory*. StoryPeople, 2007.

Baldwin, Christina. *Storycatcher*. Novato, CA: New World Library, 2007.

Carroll, Lewis. *Alice's Adventures in Wonderland & Through the Looking-Glass*. New York: Penguin, 2000.

Davis, Lennard J. "Constructing Normalcy," in *The Disability Studies Reader*. New York: Routledge, 2010.

Frank, Arthur W. *The Wounded Storyteller: Body, Illness and Ethics*. Chicago: University of Chicago Press, 1997.

Goldberg, Elkhonpn. *The Executive Brain: Frontal Lobes and the Civilized Mind*. New York: Oxford University Press, 2002.

Hutton, Jane. "Turning the Spotlight Back on the Normalising Gaze," in *The International Journal of Narrative Therapy and Community Work*, Vol. 2008, No. 1, 2008.

Leunig, Michael. *The Curly Pyjama Letters*. Melbourne: Penguin Books Australia, 2001.

Lloyd, David. *The Australian PhotoJournalist: Picturing Human Rights*. South Brisbane, Queensland: Centre for Documentary Practice, 2009.

Myerhoff, Barbara. "Life History Among the Elderly: Performance, Visibility, and Remembering," in Jay Ruby (ed.), *A Crack in the Mirror: Reflexive Perspective in Anthropology*. Philadelphia: University of Pennsylvania Press, 1982.

Ochs, Michael, Andy Selby, Jeffrey Cohen, and Molly Kaye. "In Her Eyes," recorded by Josh Groban, *Awake*, 2006.

Sacks, Oliver. *The Man Who Mistook His Wife for a Hat*. London: Picador, 1985.

Weingarten, Kaethe. "Making Sense of Illness Narratives: Braiding Theory, Practice, and the Embodied Life," in *Working With the Stories of Women's Lives*. Adelaide, South Australia: Dulwich Centre Publications, 2001.

White, Michael. *Maps of Narrative Practice*. New York: W. W. Norton, 2007.

Marie Williams has worked as a clinical social worker in health settings, nonprofit sectors, clinical education, and private practice. She is also an artist and believes in the power of creativity and story to transform. The Australian edition of Williams' book, *Green Vanilla Tea* won the national Finch Memoir Prize in 2013. Williams lives in Brisbane, Australia.

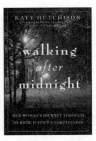
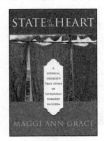
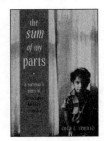
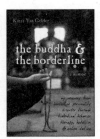
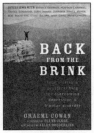
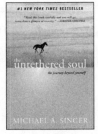
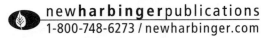